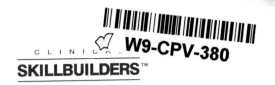

CLINICAL
SKILLBUILDERS™

W9-CPV-380

Danger Signs and Symptoms

Springhouse Corporation
Springhouse, Pennsylvania

STAFF

Executive Director, Editorial
Stanley Loeb

Editorial Director
Matthew Cahill

Clinical Director
Barbara F. McVan, RN

Art Director
John Hubbard

Senior Editor
William J. Kelly

Clinical Editors
Joanne Patzek DaCunha, RN, BS; Julie N. Tackenberg, RN, MA, CNRN

Editors
Barbara Delp, Margaret Eckman, Doris Falk, Karla Harby, Kevin Law, Elizabeth Mauro, Cheryl Namy

Copy Editors
Jane V. Cray (supervisor), Mary Hohenhaus Hardy, Amy Jirsa, Elizabeth Kiselev, Doris Weinstock

Designers
Stephanie Peters (associate art director), Julie Carlton Barlow, Beth Mead, Matie Patterson (senior designer)

Illustrators
Jean Gardner, Donna Giannola, Frank Grobelny, Robert Jackson, Debra Koenig, Robert Neumann, Judy Newhouse

Art Production
Robert Perry (manager), Heather Bernhardt, Anna Brindisi, Donald Knauss, Robert Wieder

Typography
David Kosten (director), Diane Paluba (manager), Elizabeth Bergman, Joyce Rossi Biletz, Robin Rantz, Valerie Rosenberger

Manufacturing
Deborah Meiris (manager), T.A. Landis, Jennifer Suter

Production Coordination
Aline S. Miller (manager), Laurie J. Sander

Editorial Assistants
Maree DeRosa, Beverly Lane, Mary Madden

Library of Congress
Cataloging-in-Publication Data

Danger Signs and Symptoms.

    p. cm. – (Clinical Skillbuilders™)
  Includes bibliographical references.
  Includes indexes.
    1. Emergency nursing.   2. Medical emergencies – Diagnosis. I. Springhouse Corporation. II. Series.
    [DNLM; 1. Emergencies – handbooks. 2. Emergencies – nurses' instruction.
3. Nursing Assessment – handbooks.
WY 39 D182]
RT120.E4D36 1990
616.02'5 – dc20
DNLM/DLC   90-10076
ISBN 0-87434-310-0   CIP

CONTENTS

Danger Signs and Symptoms

ADVISORY BOARD AND CONTRIBUTORS

At the time of publication, the advisors held the following positions.

Sandra G. Crandall, RN,C, MSN, CRNP
Director
Center for Nursing Excellence
Newtown, Pa.

Sandra K. Goodnough, RN, PhD
Pulmonary Clinical Nurse Specialist
Texas Woman's University
Houston

Doris A. Millam, RN, MS, CRNI
I.V. Therapy Clinician
Holy Family Hospital
Des Plaines, Ill.

Deborah Panozzo Nelson, RN, MS, CCRN
Cardiovascular Clinical Specialist
Visiting Assistant Professor
EMS Nursing Education
Purdue University, Calumet Campus
Hammond, Ind.

Marilyn Sawyer Sommers, RN, MA, CCRN
Nurse Consultant
Instructor
College of Nursing and Health
University of Cincinnati

At the time of publication, the contributors held the following positions.

Joanne Patzek DaCunha, RN, BS
Clinical Editor
Springhouse Corporation
Springhouse, Pa.

Marilyn Sawyer Sommers, RN, MA, CCRN
Nurse Consultant
Instructor
College of Nursing and Health
University of Cincinnati

FOREWORD

Today, hospitals are populated with more acutely ill patients than ever before. And that means you must assess and interpret potentially serious signs and symptoms more often than ever before. So when one of your patients develops a new sign or symptom, your first question will usually be: Does it signal an emergency?

Danger Signs and Symptoms, the latest volume in the Clinical Skillbuilders series, can help you answer that question quickly and accurately. How? By giving you the information you need to interpret 48 of the most significant signs and symptoms.

Each entry in this handy, alphabetically-arranged reference covers a sign or symptom that could indicate a life-, limb-, or organ-threatening crisis. The signs and symptoms range from the common, such as abdominal pain and headache, to the uncommon but significant, such as vision loss.

To make your job easier, each entry follows the same format. An introduction defines the sign or symptom, explains its significance, and, when appropriate, briefly discusses its pathophysiology. After that, you'll find history questions that help you explore the patient's sign or symptom in depth. Then the physical examination section tells you which assessment techniques to use. The next section correlates specific patient-history and physical examination findings with possible life-threatening causes. Each entry then ends with a listing of other possible causes.

Throughout the book, special graphic devices, or logos, call your attention to essential information about certain signs and symptoms. The *Assessment tip* logo, for instance, signals special tips or techniques that will help you zero in on your patient's problem. Whenever you see the *Emergency intervention* logo, you'll find an explanation of the steps to take when a patient needs immediate help—when he's apneic, for example. And the *Pathophysiology* logo signals an explanation of the underlying process causing a particular problem.

Following the 48 entries, you'll find a self-test. Taking it will help you measure what you've learned and further build your skills.

With all of this practical and valuable information packed into one volume, *Danger Signs and Symptoms* is guaranteed to help virtually any nurse. If you're a student, a recent graduate, or a nurse new to a clinical area, this book can serve as your private mentor. If you're an experienced nurse, it will help you sharpen your skills and give you new insights.

Novice and veteran nurses alike agree we can't be too prepared for our patients. They deserve nurses who can interpret their signs and symptoms accurately and intervene appropriately. Many books promise to help us do this. *Danger Signs and Symptoms* delivers.

Nancy M. Holloway, RN, MSN, CCRN, CEN
Critical Care Educator
Nancy Holloway and Associates
Oakland, California

INTRODUCTION

When your patient tells you he feels chest pain, he may be suffering an acute myocardial infarction . . . or he may only have gastric reflux.

How do you know? Well, you can begin by recognizing an often-overlooked fact: that the cause of chest pain, or any other potential danger sign or symptom, won't be apparent until you assess the patient. Even if you know his history, you can't assume that his current symptom is related to his existing medical problem.

The signs and symptoms in this book *may* indicate life-, limb-, or organ-threatening emergencies. But in most cases, you won't know if they do until you ask appropriate history questions and examine the patient.

This book tells you which questions to ask and which assessment procedures to perform. What's more, it helps you correlate your assessment findings so you can determine whether the sign or symptom actually signals an emergency.

Identifying a danger sign or symptom

You may detect a potential danger sign or symptom in one of two ways. While assessing a patient, you may identify a sign — a weak pulse, for example. But more commonly, you'll learn of a potential danger sign or symptom when your patient complains about it. He may tell you, for instance, that his heart feels as though it's racing or that he's short of breath.

When a patient reports such a symptom, you may feel that you need to intervene immediately or call the patient's doctor. But almost always you should perform a quick, thorough assessment first. In many cases, the sign or symptom will prove to be a normal variation or an effect of a less serious or a chronic disorder.

How do you determine whether a sign or symptom signals an emergency? By using a consistent, systematic approach to gather and evaluate information. Each time you assess a patient, for example, you'll need to determine the relationship of his current problem to other signs and symptoms and monitor him for any changes. Only then can you narrow the list of possible causes and determine whether the patient truly needs immediate intervention.

Quick assessment

What about time constraints? In a potential life-, limb- or organ-threatening situation, isn't assessment severely limited by the need for immediate intervention? In some situations, yes. But in most cases, nursing and medical interventions can wait until you complete a quick, systematic assessment.

Keep in mind that collecting appropriate assessment data shouldn't take long. Usually, you can collect history information and perform the physical examination at the same time. In an emergency that poses an imminent threat, you may assess and intervene simultaneously. For example, if you suspect an airway obstruction, you should assess the patient's airway, remove the obstruction, then recheck breathing and circulation — all in rapid succession.

Even when you're faced with a danger sign that typically requires immediate intervention—apnea, for example—you should assess first. Suppose on a routine nighttime check of a patient, you detect a respiratory rate of less than 6 breaths/minute. If you immediately intervene without further assessing the patient, you might perform unnecessary cardiopulmonary resuscitation on a patient who has chronic uncomplicated sleep apnea or a patient who is a yoga enthusiast and has learned to decrease his respiratory rate during sleep. Even if you have reason to suspect a life-threatening situation, you need to determine whether the patient is responsive, check his airway for obstruction, and assess his respirations and pulse. In some cases, you'd have to quickly assess his neurologic status to determine if ineffective ventilations result from a neuromuscular deficit.

Collecting assessment data

As you know, nursing assessment includes gathering a health history and a physical examination. For each danger sign and symptom in this book, you'll find history questions you can use to focus your investigation. You'll also find a description of the assessment procedures you should use to obtain information as quickly as possible.

Health history
Usually, you'll obtain information from the patient, but not always. In certain situations—for example, if the patient is unconscious—you may have to obtain information from a family member, a witness, or an emergency medical technician. A hospitalized patient may have significant history information recorded in his medical record.

Chief complaint. Start your investigation by finding out some basic information about the chief sign or symptom. Ask when it began, how severe it is, and how long it's lasted. Also, find out whether the patient ever had the sign or symptom before. If so, what treatment did he receive? Ask if anything aggravates or alleviates the sign or symptom.

When evaluating this information, remember that a patient's complaints are *subjective,* based on his perception of how the episode threatens his life or health. Several factors contribute to this perception, including the patient's previous experience with the symptom. A person who's experiencing dyspnea for the first time may describe the episode as severe, but someone with chronic obstructive pulmonary disease (COPD) might describe a similar episode as mild. That's because the person who's never experienced dyspnea has nothing to compare it with and may assume the worst, whereas the COPD patient may have experienced similar episodes and trusts that treatment will alleviate the symptom.

Other factors that can influence the perception of a symptom include:
• anxiety and fear. When your patient is anxious or afraid, his response will usually be exaggerated.
• lack of external stimuli. Pain commonly worsens at night because the patient has no distractions. Thus, he focuses solely on what he's feeling.
• cultural influences. Persons of certain cultural backgrounds tend to respond emotionally to a change in their health, whereas persons from other cultures may remain stoic despite severe symptoms.

• knowledge of another's bad experience. If a friend or family member had a similar symptom and experienced a bad outcome, the patient may assume the same thing will happen to him.

Further investigation. Besides investigating the patient's chief complaint, also ask about any other signs or symptoms he's experiencing. Explore the characteristics of each as you did for the chief complaint. Also, determine the relationship of the associated sign or symptom to the chief complaint. For instance, did it precede, coincide with, or follow the onset of the chief complaint?

Then investigate whether the chief sign or symptom is linked to a recent episode. For example, has the patient been exposed to toxic substances or allergens or eaten a particular food? Maybe he's experienced trauma. Or perhaps he's undergone a therapeutic procedure, such as subclavian catheterization or mechanical ventilation.

Also explore any existing or past medical conditions that may help reveal the cause of the chief complaint. Ask about the family history too. As appropriate and as time permits, ask about occupational and environmental conditions, identifying any circumstances that could pose a health risk.

Finally, be sure to obtain a medication history. Cover all types of drugs: prescription medications, over-the-counter products, and such drugs as alcohol, caffeine, and illicit mind- and mood-altering substances. Investigate how often the patient takes each drug. This will help you detect any misuse or abuse and determine the last time he took each drug. Don't forget to ask about vitamin use. Many patients don't consider vitamins to be drugs. But excessive dosages can cause toxic effects. Vitamin A toxicity, for example, can produce pseudotumor cerebri, marked by signs of increased intracranial pressure.

Physical examination

For every patient, you'll perform an initial physical examination based on the health history findings. The information you gather during this examination will help you further narrow your list of suspected causes.

The examination also provides baseline information for later comparison. After the initial physical examination, you should perform an ongoing assessment to detect and evaluate changes — no matter how seemingly minor.

Sometimes, the presence of a sign or symptom doesn't mean as much as a change from the baseline. For instance, a blood pressure reading of 90/50 mm Hg may not be significant if it's a patient's normal reading. Even if a blood pressure reading is low for a particular patient, it may not be significant if he's asymptomatic. In this instance, you'd have to monitor for a further drop in blood pressure and for associated signs and symptoms.

Examination sequence. Usually, your physical examination will follow the standard sequence: inspection, palpation, percussion, and auscultation. But if you suspect an abdominal problem, you should auscultate the abdomen before palpating and percussing it. This alternative sequence ensures that you don't change the frequency and intensity of bowel sounds before you auscultate them.

Begin your examination by carefully observing the patient's overall appearance, focusing on areas implicated by the health history findings.

Example: For an unconscious patient with a history of diabetes mellitus, you'd smell his breath for a fruity odor. If you note such an odor, he may have diabetic ketoacidosis—a life-threatening condition requiring immediate intervention.

Continue your physical examination using palpation, percussion, and auscultation techniques. Systematically assess the appropriate body systems and areas, checking for any abnormalities that may correlate with the patient's chief complaint and accompanying symptoms—and help point to the underlying cause.

Identifying the cause
Following the section on the physical examination, you'll find a listing of possible life-, limb-, or organ-threatening disorders that may cause the danger sign or symptom. Under each possible cause, you'll see a discussion of the sign's or symptom's characteristics—onset, severity, duration, and so on—and of important accompanying signs and symptoms that you'd likely detect during your assessment. You'll also find a listing of other possible causes—ones that may not require immediate intervention. By using these lists, you may be able to quickly identify the cause of a patient's problem and thus determine appropriate nursing interventions and anticipate medical interventions.

The next time you're faced with a potential danger sign or symptom, use this systematic approach. Remember, your main focus is to collect the essential assessment information quickly. Only then can you intervene appropriately—and perhaps preserve organ function, maintain limb integrity, or even save a patient's life.

DANGER SIGNS AND SYMPTOMS

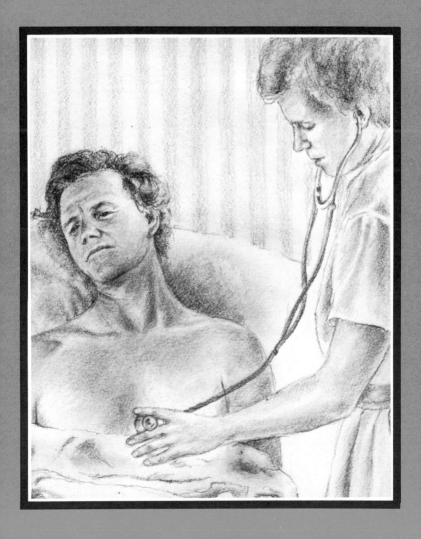

Abdominal pain

Abdominal pain may originate in the abdominopelvic viscera, the parietal peritoneum, or the capsules of the liver, kidney, or spleen. The pain may be acute or chronic, diffuse or localized. Visceral pain develops slowly into a dull ache that's poorly localized in the epigastric, periumbilical, or lower midabdominal region. By contrast, somatic pain develops quickly after an insult and is sharp, more intense, and well localized. Moving or coughing aggravates this pain.

Sometimes, abdominal pain is referred from another site that has the same or a similar nerve supply. This sharp, well-localized pain of the skin or deeper tissues may be accompanied by skin hyperesthesia and muscle hyperalgesia (see *Understanding types of abdominal pain*).

Abdominal pain can be produced by several mechanisms: stretching of or tension on the gut wall, traction on the peritoneum or mesentery, vigorous intestinal contraction, inflammation, ischemia, or sensory nerve irritation. Persistent pain may result from blood in the peritoneal cavity, organ perforation, ischemia, or inflammation. Intermittent cramps may indicate an obstruction of a hollow organ.

History questions
Explore the patient's problem by asking appropriate questions from this section.

• Find out when the patient's pain began. Did it start suddenly or gradually? Where exactly is the pain? Is it localized or diffuse?

• Have the patient describe the pain in detail. Is it dull, sharp, cramping, colicky, or a feeling of tenderness? Does the intensity vary? Find out if the pain radiates to other areas, such as the chest or back. Is it constant or intermittent? If it's intermittent, how long does a typical episode last? Determine if the pain gets better or worse when the patient changes position, moves, walks, exerts himself, coughs, vomits, eats, or has a bowel movement.

• Does the patient have a fever? If so, did it begin before or after the pain started? Is he experiencing dyspnea or tachypnea? Find out if his appetite has changed. Has he felt nauseated and been vomiting? If so, when did he start vomiting and how often does it occur? Ask if he's been constipated, had diarrhea, or noticed changes in stool consistency. Determine when he had his last bowel movement. Has he experienced urinary frequency or urgency? Pain when urinating? Is his urine cloudy or pink?

• If the patient is a woman of childbearing age, ask the date of her last menses. Has her menstrual pattern changed? Could she be pregnant? Is she having vaginal bleeding? What about dyspareunia?

• Has the patient had headaches recently?

• Find out if he's traveled to a foreign country recently or if he could have eaten or drank contaminated food.

• Ask if the patient has a history of medical problems, such as adrenal disease, dyspnea, heart disease, diabetes mellitus, recent infection, hemoglobinopathies, chronic leukemia, or blunt trauma to the abdomen, flank, or chest. Has he had radiation therapy or abdominal surgery?

Understanding types of abdominal pain

AFFECTED ORGAN	VISCERAL PAIN	PARIETAL PAIN	REFERRED PAIN
Stomach	Midepigastrium	Midepigastrium and left upper quadrant	Shoulders
Small intestine	Periumbilical area	Over affected site	Midback (rare)
Appendix	Periumbilical area	Right lower quadrant	Right lower quadrant
Proximal colon	Periumbilical area and right flank for ascending colon	Over affected site	Right lower quadrant and back (rare)
Distal colon	Hypogastrium and left flank for descending colon	Over affected site	Left lower quadrant and back (rare)
Gallbladder	Midepigastrium	Right upper quadrant	Right subscapular area
Ureters	Costovertebral angle	Over affected site	Groin; scrotum in men, labia in women (rare)
Pancreas	Midepigastrium and left upper quadrant	Midepigastrium and left upper quadrant	Back and left shoulder
Ovaries, fallopian tubes, and uterus	Hypogastrium and groin	Over affected site	Inner thighs

• Does the patient have a history of a disorder that would predispose him to emboli? Such disorders include mitral stenosis, infective endocarditis, atrial fibrillation, microthrombi in the left ventricle, rheumatic heart disease, thrombophlebitis of the inferior vena cava or lower legs, congestive heart failure (CHF), or a recent myocardial infarction (MI). Does he have a history of a disorder that can narrow the arterial lumen — periarteritis, sickle cell disease, scleroderma, atherosclerosis, or arteriolar nephrosclerosis, for example? Has he recently undergone a urinary tract procedure or surgery?

• Determine if the patient has a history of I.V. drug or alcohol abuse. Has he undergone transfusions of blood or blood products? If the patient is a male, has he engaged in homosexual activity?

• What drugs has the patient taken? Note particularly any drugs that may cause pancreatitis, such as azathioprine, ethacrynic acid, furosemide, opiates, corticosteroids, oral contraceptives, sulfonamides, and thiazide diuretics. Also note any drugs that may produce CHF, such as beta blockers, corticosteroids, or biological response modifiers; hepatitis, such as oral contraceptives; or MI, such as cocaine.

Physical examination

Base your assessment of the patient on the health history information you've collected. Assess his abdomen, making sure you auscultate before palpating and percussing. Using this alternative sequence ensures that you don't affect the frequency or intensity of bowel sounds before you assess them.

Inspection. Observe the patient's skin for diaphoresis and jaundice, indicating hepatic or biliary obstruction. Also look for discoloration and coolness or edema of the arms and legs, indicating decreased oxygenation or cardiac output. Check for poor skin turgor. Inspect the skin of the abdomen and chest for signs of trauma, such as lacerations, puncture wounds, or ecchymoses. Also, look for a bluish discoloration around the umbilicus (Cullen's sign) and around the flank area (Turner's sign), which can indicate blunt trauma.

After observing for abdominal distention, obtain and record a baseline measurement of abdominal girth at the umbilicus. Later increases can indicate bleeding. Then observe the abdomen for visible peristaltic waves.

Inspect for neck vein distention. Then check the rate and depth of the patient's respirations. See if he's having trouble breathing, and observe for irregular rhythms, such as tachypnea or Kussmaul's respirations. Assess his level of consciousness. During subsequent examinations, check if any significant changes have occurred.

Note urine odor and color.

Auscultation. Next, auscultate for bowel sounds, noting whether they're high-pitched and tinkling, hyperactive, or absent. (See *Locating abdominal sounds*.)

Then listen to the heart rate and check for abnormal heart sounds. Auscultate the lungs for crackles and decreased or absent breath sounds. Monitor the patient's blood pressure and pulse pressure.

Palpation. As you systematically palpate the entire abdominal, pelvic, and epigastric areas, note any masses, rigidity, tenderness, tenderness with guarding, rebound tenderness, or enlarged organs (see *Assessing for rebound tenderness,* page 6). To determine kidney size, palpate the flank. Then check peripheral pulses for rate, rhythm, and intensity.

Percussion. After that, percuss over each abdominal quadrant, noting the percussion sounds as well as any tenderness or increased pain. Dull percussion sounds indicate free fluid; hollow percussion sounds indicate air. Percuss over the costovertebral angle (CVA) to elicit any pain.

Life-threatening causes

Your assessment may lead you to suspect one or more of the following.

Abdominal aortic aneurysm (dissecting). Constant, dull upper abdominal pain radiating to the low back often accompanies rapid aneurysmal enlargement and may herald rupture (see *Abdominal pain: Linking location and cause,* page 7). The pain may worsen when the patient lies down and subside when he leans forward or sits up. On palpation, you may note an epigastric mass that pulsates before rupture but not after it and tenderness over the aneurysm. You may also auscultate a systolic bruit over the aneurysm.

Locating abdominal sounds

When you auscultate the abdomen, you'll find that particular sounds are clearer in certain areas than in others. This illustration shows you the best place to listen for various sounds.

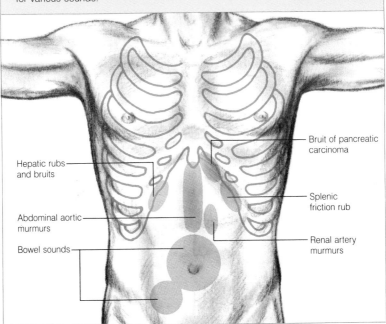

Hepatic rubs and bruits

Abdominal aortic murmurs

Bowel sounds

Bruit of pancreatic carcinoma

Splenic friction rub

Renal artery murmurs

Other findings may include mottled skin below the waist, absent femoral and pedal pulses, lower blood pressure in the legs than in the arms, mild to moderate abdominal tenderness with guarding, increasing abdominal girth, and abdominal rigidity. Signs of hypovolemic shock — tachycardia, tachypnea, hypotension, and cool, clammy skin — may appear. The patient may have a history of atherosclerosis.

Abdominal trauma. The patient may have generalized or localized abdominal pain along with abdominal ecchymoses, Cullen's or Turner's sign, abdominal tenderness, or vomiting. If he's hemorrhaging into the peritoneal cavity, you may note dullness on percussion, increasing abdominal girth, and abdominal rigidity. You may hear hollow bowel sounds if an abdominal organ is perforated, or bowel sounds may be absent. If you hear them in the chest cavity, the patient probably has a diaphragmatic tear.

Adrenal crisis. Severe abdominal pain along with nausea, vomiting, weakness, anorexia, and fever usually occur in this disorder. The patient may have a previous history of adrenal disease, signs of preexisting adrenal disease, a recent history

Assessing for rebound tenderness

To check for rebound tenderness, press deeply and gently into the patient's abdomen with your fingertips.

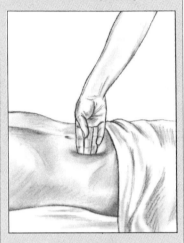

Then, rapidly withdraw your fingertips. If the patient feels pain, the problem may be peritoneal irritation—possibly the result of appendicitis.

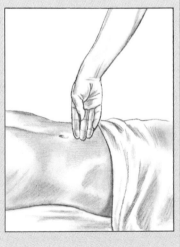

of headaches (suggesting impending adrenal crisis), or a history of noncompliance with a corticosteroid regimen. Excessive corticosteroid use can trigger an adrenal crisis.

Appendicitis. In this disorder, a dull discomfort or severe pain in the epigastric or umbilical region typically follows anorexia, nausea, vomiting, and diarrhea or constipation. Pain localizes at McBurney's point in the right lower quadrant. This may be accompanied by abdominal rigidity, increasing tenderness (especially over McBurney's point), rebound tenderness, and retractions on respiration. The onset may be sudden, or the patient may have milder and flulike symptoms for a few hours or days before he seeks medical attention. (For more information, see *Identifying causes of referred pain*, page 8.)

Congestive heart failure. Right upper quadrant pain commonly accompanies the hallmarks of this disorder: neck vein distention, dyspnea, bibasilar crackles, tachycardia, and peripheral edema. Other findings may include tachypnea, orthopnea, normal or low blood pressure, nausea, vomiting, dependent edema, ascites, hepatomegaly, productive cough, cool extremities, cold intolerance, and circumoral and nail bed cyanosis. On auscultation, you may hear an atrial or a ventricular gallop. The patient's medical history may include heart disease, edema, weight gain, fatigue, diaphoresis, or progressive dyspnea. Or this may be the first episode of noncompliance with a medication regimen. The patient's medication history may include use of amiodarone, carbamazepine, encainide, flecainide, recombinant interferon alfa-2a, recombinant interleukin-2,

Abdominal pain: Linking location and cause

This illustration shows you what pain in different abdominal areas may mean. Life-threatening causes appear in italics.

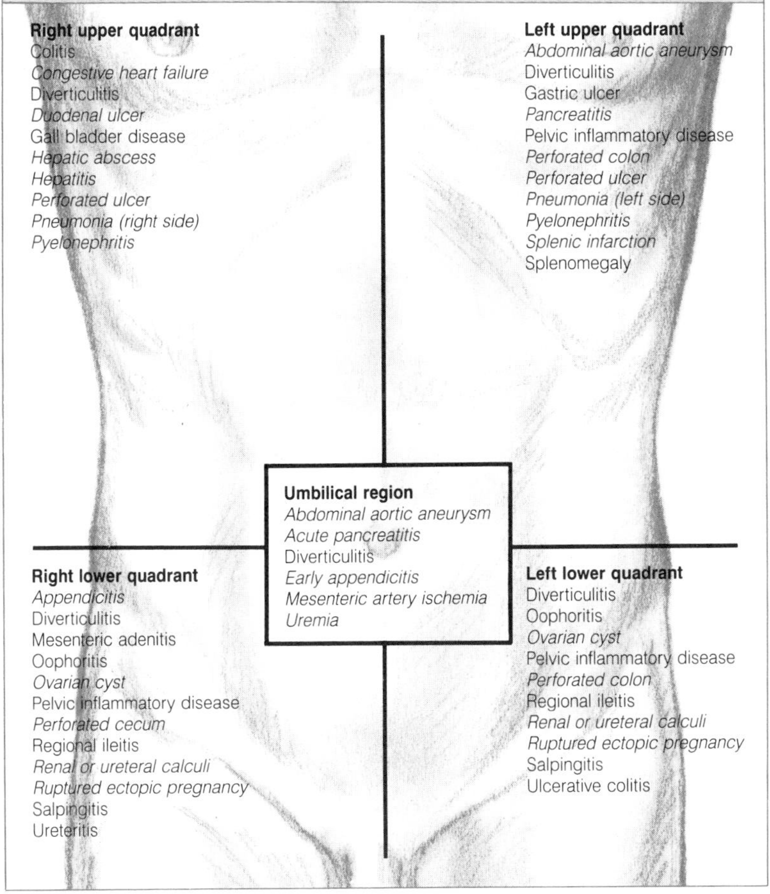

Right upper quadrant
Colitis
Congestive heart failure
Diverticulitis
Duodenal ulcer
Gall bladder disease
Hepatic abscess
Hepatitis
Perforated ulcer
Pneumonia (right side)
Pyelonephritis

Left upper quadrant
Abdominal aortic aneurysm
Diverticulitis
Gastric ulcer
Pancreatitis
Pelvic inflammatory disease
Perforated colon
Perforated ulcer
Pneumonia (left side)
Pyelonephritis
Splenic infarction
Splenomegaly

Umbilical region
Abdominal aortic aneurysm
Acute pancreatitis
Diverticulitis
Early appendicitis
Mesenteric artery ischemia
Uremia

Right lower quadrant
Appendicitis
Diverticulitis
Mesenteric adenitis
Oophoritis
Ovarian cyst
Pelvic inflammatory disease
Perforated cecum
Regional ileitis
Renal or ureteral calculi
Ruptured ectopic pregnancy
Salpingitis
Ureteritis

Left lower quadrant
Diverticulitis
Oophoritis
Ovarian cyst
Pelvic inflammatory disease
Perforated colon
Regional ileitis
Renal or ureteral calculi
Ruptured ectopic pregnancy
Salpingitis
Ulcerative colitis

angiotensin-converting enzyme inhibitors, beta blockers, calcium channel blockers, corticosteroids, or nonsteroidal anti-inflammatory drugs — any of which can cause CHF.

Diabetic ketoacidosis. Rarely, a patient with diabetic ketoacidosis (DKA) has severe, sharp, shooting, and girdling abdominal pain for several days. This pain may be accompanied by polydipsia, polyuria, polyphagia, weight loss, and weakness. Other signs and symptoms include fruity breath odor, hypotension, flushed face, decreased pulse pressure, a weak and rapid pulse, Kussmaul's respirations,

Identifying causes of referred pain

These illustrations show you the causes of referred abdominal pain.

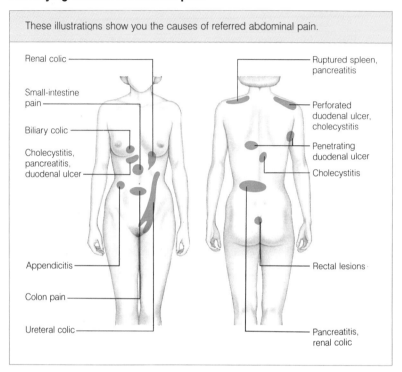

Renal colic

Small-intestine pain

Biliary colic

Cholecystitis, pancreatitis, duodenal ulcer

Appendicitis

Colon pain

Ureteral colic

Ruptured spleen, pancreatitis

Perforated duodenal ulcer, cholecystitis

Penetrating duodenal ulcer

Cholecystitis

Rectal lesions

Pancreatitis, renal colic

nausea, vomiting, and poor skin turgor. Seizures and stupor that may progress to coma result from sodium and extracellular fluid loss. The patient may have diabetes mellitus and may have failed to comply with his medication or diet regimen.

Ectopic pregnancy. Lower abdominal pain may be sharp, dull, or cramping and either constant or intermittent. The pain may be accompanied by vaginal bleeding, nausea, vomiting, urinary frequency, a tender adnexal mass, breast tenderness or enlargement, and a 1- to 2-month history of amenorrhea after sexual intercourse. (If your patient is an adolescent, keep in mind that she may not admit to having had intercourse, especially if her parent is present during the examination.)

Rupture of the fallopian tube produces sharp lower abdominal pain, which may radiate to the shoulders and neck and become extreme on cervical or adnexal palpation. Signs of shock, such as pallor, tachycardia, and hypotension, may also appear.

Hepatic abscess. Right upper quadrant tenderness is the most important finding in this rare disorder, which also commonly produces steady, severe abdominal pain in the right upper quadrant or midepigastrium. Other signs and symptoms include anorexia, diarrhea, nausea, fever, diaphoresis, and, infrequently, vomiting. The patient's recent history may include bacteremia, particularly from cholangitis; foreign travel; or ingestion of contaminated food.

Hepatitis. Liver enlargement from any type of hepatitis will cause discomfort or dull pain and tenderness in the right upper quadrant. Associated signs and symptoms may include dark urine, clay-colored stools, nausea, vomiting, anorexia, jaundice, and pruritus. The patient may have ingested contaminated food, particularly shellfish, or used a drug that can cause hepatitis, such as a sulfonamide, methyldopa, or isotretinoin. His history may also include I.V. drug abuse, a blood transfusion, or male homosexual activity.

Intestinal obstruction. In this disorder, short episodes of intense, colicky, cramping pain alternate with pain-free periods. Accompanying signs and symptoms may include abdominal distention, tenderness, and guarding; tympany; visible peristaltic waves; obstipation; and pain-induced agitation. You may note high-pitched, tinkling, or hyperactive bowel sounds proximal to the obstruction and lower-pitched, hypoactive, or absent bowel sounds distal to it. In jejunal and duodenal obstruction, nausea and bilious vomiting occur early. In distal small-bowel or large-bowel obstruction, nausea and vomiting are often feculent. Complete obstruction causes absent bowel sounds. Hypotension, tachycardia, tachypnea, and cool, clammy skin indicate hypovolemic shock. The patient may have a history of

bloody stool. Or he may have had abdominal radiation therapy or surgery that can cause adhesions.

Mesenteric artery ischemia. The patient will have severe, constant, and diffuse abdominal pain preceded by 2 to 3 days of colicky periumbilical pain and diarrhea. Associated findings include vomiting, anorexia, and alternating periods of diarrhea (which may be bloody) and constipation. In the late stages, extreme abdominal tenderness with rigidity may develop. Hypotension, tachycardia, tachypnea, and cool, clammy skin indicate hypovolemic or septic shock. The patient's history may include a recent episode of hypoperfusion, such as hypotension, CHF, or cardiac dysrhythmias.

Myocardial infarction. In this disorder, the patient may have substernal ischemic chest pain unrelieved by nitroglycerin. This pain may radiate to the abdomen, left arm, jaw, neck, or shoulder blades. Accompanying signs and symptoms include pallor, weakness, diaphoresis, dizziness, nausea, vomiting, anxiety, dyspnea, and a feeling of impending doom. Hypotension, tachycardia, tachypnea, and cool, clammy skin may indicate cardiogenic shock. The patient may develop hypotension or hypertension, an atrial gallop, murmurs, a pericardial friction rub, and crackles. His history may include heart disease, hypertension, or hypercholesterolemia. Or this episode may be the first indication of a heart problem. The patient's medication history may include the use of drugs, such as dextrothyroxine, extramustine phosphate sodium, and recombinant interleukin-2, that can lead to an MI. Or he may have taken cocaine.

Ovarian cyst. In this disorder, torsion or hemorrhage may cause pain and tenderness in the right or left lower abdominal quadrant. Sharp and severe if the patient suddenly stands or stoops, the pain becomes brief and intermittent if the torsion corrects itself, or dull and diffuse after several hours if it doesn't. Accompanying signs and symptoms may include a slight fever, mild nausea and vomiting, abdominal tenderness, a palpable mass, and possibly amenorrhea. With large cysts, abdominal distention may develop. Peritoneal irritation or rupture and peritonitis also cause high fever, abdominal rigidity, and severe nausea and vomiting. The patient's history usually isn't significant.

Pancreatitis. The characteristic symptom of this disorder is fulminating, continuous upper abdominal pain that may radiate to both flanks and to the back. To relieve this pain, the patient may bend forward, draw his knees to his chest, or move restlessly about. Abdominal tenderness, nausea, vomiting, fever, pallor, tachycardia, and, in some patients, abdominal rigidity, abdominal distention, rebound tenderness, and hypoactive bowel sounds may also occur. Turner's or Cullen's sign indicates hemorrhagic pancreatitis.

The patient's history may include alcohol abuse, gallbladder disease, diabetes mellitus, trauma, or a scorpion bite. Or he may have taken a drug that can cause pancreatitis — a thiazide diuretic, for example.

Perforated ulcer. Sudden, severe, prostrating epigastric pain may radiate through the patient's abdomen to the back. Other signs and symptoms include boardlike abdominal rigidity, tenderness with guarding, generalized rebound tenderness, absent bowel sounds, grunting and shallow respirations, and fever. Hypotension, tachycardia, tachypnea, and cool, clammy skin indicate hypovolemic shock. The patient's history may include a gastric or duodenal ulcer or complaints of frequent stomach upset, heartburn, or epigastric pain.

Peritonitis. A patient may experience sudden, severe pain that's either diffuse or localized in the area of the underlying disorder. With appendicitis, for example, the pain will occur in the right lower quadrant; with an ectopic pregnancy or ovarian cyst, it'll occur in the lower pelvic region. When the patient moves, the pain worsens.

In some cases, the original pain may change before the onset of the current symptoms. For instance, if the appendix ruptures, the pain may subside for a short while. Or if an ovarian cyst or fallopian tube ruptures, the pain may suddenly become intense. The patient also may have fever; chills; nausea; vomiting; hypoactive or absent bowel sounds; abdominal tenderness, distention, and rigidity; rebound tenderness and guarding; and hyperalgesia. Hypotension, tachycardia, tachypnea, and cool, clammy skin indicate septic shock. The patient may have a history of abdominal pain and flulike symptoms for a few hours or days before seeking medical attention.

Pneumonia. Lower lobe pneumonia can cause pleuritic chest pain and referred, severe upper abdominal pain, tenderness, and rigidity — all of which diminish on inspiration. Other signs and symptoms include fever, shaking chills, tachypnea, myalgia, fatigue, anorexia, diaphoresis, headache, and dyspnea. The patient may also have a dry, hacking cough or a cough that produces blood-tinged or rusty sputum, which may be foul-smelling. On auscultation, you may detect decreased breath sounds, crackles, rhonchi, whispered pectoriloquy, or tachycardia. The patient's history may include exposure to someone with pneumonia or to hazardous fumes or air pollution. He may also have chronic obstructive pulmonary disease or a history of smoking.

Pneumothorax. Sudden, sharp chest pain, dyspnea, and cyanosis are the cardinal signs of pneumothorax. The patient may also feel referred pain across the upper abdomen and costal margin. Characteristically, the pain strikes suddenly and worsens with deep inspiration or movement. Accompanying signs and symptoms include anxiety, restlessness, decreased or absent breath sounds, decreased vocal fremitus, hyperresonance and tympany over the affected area, subcutaneous crepitation, asymmetrical chest expansion, accessory muscle use, a nonproductive cough, tachypnea, and tachycardia. Usually, the patient has a history of trauma, chronic obstructive pulmonary disease, subclavian vein cannulation, lung cancer, or mechanical ventilation under pressure. But pneumothorax can occur spontaneously.

Pyelonephritis (acute). Progressive upper quadrant pain on one or both sides, flank pain, and CVA tenderness characterize this disorder. Pain may radiate to the lower midabdominal region or the groin. Other signs and symptoms may include abdominal and back tenderness, high fever, shaking chills, nausea,

vomiting, hematuria, dysuria, tenesmus, and urinary frequency and urgency. The patient's urine may smell like ammonia. His history may include an infection (most commonly of the urinary tract), a recent invasive procedure, neurogenic bladder, diabetes mellitus, or compromised renal function. Women who are sexually active or pregnant are susceptible to this disorder.

Renal calculi. Depending on the location of the calculi, the patient may feel severe abdominal or back pain. The classic symptom, however, is severe, colicky pain that travels from the CVA to the flank, the suprapubic region, and the external genitalia. The pain may be dull and constant or excruciating. Pain-induced agitation, nausea, vomiting, abdominal distention, fever, chills, and urinary urgency may occur. The patient's history isn't usually significant.

Renal infarction. With this disorder, a patient may have severe, continuous upper abdominal pain, flank pain, and CVA tenderness. Other signs and symptoms include anorexia, nausea, vomiting, hypoactive bowel sounds, and fever. Percussing the CVA will elicit pain. The patient may have a history of disorders predisposing him to emboli, such as mitral stenosis or atrial fibrillation, or disorders that narrow the arterial lumen, such as atherosclerosis.

Splenic infarction. This disorder produces fulminating pain in the left upper quadrant along with chest pain that may worsen on inspiration. In many cases, the pain radiates to the left shoulder. The patient may splint the left diaphragm and guard his abdomen. You may note a splenic friction rub. The patient may have a history of hemoglobinopathies or chronic leukemia, which are predisposing factors.

Uremia. Characterized by generalized or periumbilical pain that shifts and varies in intensity, this disorder causes diverse GI symptoms, including nausea, vomiting, anorexia, and diarrhea. Abdominal tenderness that changes in location and intensity may occur, along with visual disturbances, bleeding, headache, a decreased level of consciousness, irritability, vertigo, and oliguria or anuria. A patient with uremia may have a history of renal disease.

Other causes
Abdominal pain also results from conditions that may not require immediate intervention.

Disorders. Abdominal pain may result from anxiety, nausea, or vomiting. It may also result from abdominal cancer, cholecystitis, cholelithiasis, cirrhosis, Crohn's disease, cystitis, diverticulitis, duodenal ulcer, endometriosis, gastric ulcer, gastritis, gastroenteritis, hepatic amebiasis, herpes zoster, ileitis, and cellular toxicity caused by an insect bite. What's more, abdominal pain may stem from irritable bowel syndrome, lactose intolerance, mesenteric adenitis, oophoritis, chronic pancreatitis, pelvic inflammatory disease, pleurisy, prostatitis, salpingitis, sickle cell crisis, systemic lupus erythematosus, ulcerative colitis, and ureteritis.

Drugs. Salicylates and nonsteroidal anti-inflammatory drugs commonly cause burning, gnawing pain in the left upper quadrant or the epigastric area. Many other drugs

cause abdominal pain. These include the anthelmintics, antilipemics, antimalarials, cephalosporins, cholinergics, laxatives, progestins, and calcium and potassium salts.

Other drugs that may produce abdominal pain are cinoxacin, clofazimine, cyclobenzaprine, dantrolene, dapsone, diphenoxylate with atropine, disopyramide, erythromycin, ethambutol, fenfluramine, flecainide, imipramine, ketoconazole, loperamide, maprotiline, methyldopa, methylphenidate, nalidixic acid, naltrexone, nitroprusside, nortriptyline, para-aminosalicylate sodium, pemoline, protriptyline, quinidine, tranylcypromine, trimethadione, and trimipramine.

Abdominal rigidity

Detected by palpation, abdominal rigidity is characterized by inflexibility or abnormal muscle tension. Rigidity may be either voluntary or involuntary. Voluntary rigidity (or guarding) results from a patient's fear or nervousness as you palpate his abdomen. Involuntary rigidity, on the other hand, may indicate a potentially life-threatening disorder, such as peritoneal irritation or inflammation. With children, you may have trouble distinguishing voluntary from involuntary rigidity because of the fear caused by the associated pain.

History questions
Explore the patient's problem by asking appropriate questions from this section.
● Does the patient have abdominal pain? If so, did it start at the same time as the abdominal rigidity? Is the pain localized or generalized?

Does it radiate? Has it moved? Ask if the rigidity or pain gets worse or better when the patient inhales, coughs, changes position, walks, vomits, or has a bowel movement.

• Does the patient's recent history include anorexia, vomiting, diarrhea, or constipation? What about fever or flulike symptoms? Has he been bitten by an insect or spider? If not, ask if he's been in a situation where he could've been bitten.

• Has the patient ever had abdominal trauma, cardiovascular disease, diabetes mellitus, gallbladder disease, or peptic ulcer disease? Does he have a history of smoking or alcohol abuse?

• Is the patient taking any drugs that could cause pancreatitis, such as azathioprine, ethacrynic acid, or furosemide? What about opiates, oral contraceptives, sulfonamides, thiazide diuretics, or corticosteroids?

Physical examination

Base your assessment of the patient on the health history information you've collected. Assess his abdomen, making sure you auscultate before palpating and percussing. Using this alternative sequence ensures that you don't affect the frequency or intensity of bowel sounds before you assess them.

Inspection. Observe for peristaltic waves, which you may be able to see in thin patients, and check for a distended bowel loop. Then inspect the skin below the waist for mottling, which may result from poor circulation. Look for poor skin turgor and dry mucous membranes — indications of dehydration.

Take a baseline measurement of the patient's abdominal girth at the umbilicus. A later increase may indicate bleeding.

Observe the rate and depth of his respirations. Does he have difficulty breathing or an abnormal respiratory pattern?

Auscultation. Listen for bowel sounds, noting whether they're absent, hypoactive, or hyperactive. To distinguish between hypoactive and absent bowel sounds, listen over the same spot for at least 5 minutes. Then place the bell of your stethoscope over the abdominal aorta to auscultate for abdominal bruits. Monitor the patient's blood pressure and pulse pressure.

Palpation. Use light palpation to locate abdominal rigidity, determining whether it's localized or generalized. Evaluate the severity. Be sure to distinguish between voluntary and involuntary rigidity (see *Distinguishing voluntary from involuntary rigidity,* page 14). Also, check for abdominal masses, especially ones that pulsate. Remember that palpating with cold hands causes the abdomen to contract, interfering with your assessment. Check peripheral pulses for rate, rhythm, and intensity. Then palpate the femoral and pedal pulses, and note if either is absent on one or both sides.

Percussion. As you lightly percuss each abdominal quadrant, check for pain, tenderness, and abnormal sounds.

Life-threatening causes

Your assessment may lead you to suspect one or more of the following.

Abdominal aortic aneurysm (dissecting). A patient with this disorder may have abdominal rigidity accompanied by dull, constant upper abdominal pain. This pain, which

Distinguishing voluntary from involuntary rigidity

When assessing abdominal rigidity, you need to determine whether it's voluntary or involuntary. This comparison will help you do just that.

Voluntary rigidity is:
- usually symmetrical
- more noticeable on inspiration (because expiration relaxes muscles)
- eased by relaxation techniques, such as positioning the patient comfortably and talking to him in a calm, soothing voice
- painless when the patient sits up using only his abdominal muscles.

Involuntary rigidity is:
- usually asymmetrical
- equally noticeable on inspiration and expiration
- unaffected by relaxation techniques
- painful when the patient sits up using only his abdominal muscles.

may radiate to the low back, results from a rapidly enlarging aneurysm that's ready to rupture. The patient may feel more pain when he lies down and less when he sits up or leans forward. You may palpate a pulsating epigastric mass and auscultate a systolic bruit over the abdominal aorta. After the rupture, the pulsating stops.

Other signs and symptoms may include mottled skin below the waist, absent femoral and pedal pulses, blood pressure that's lower in the legs than in the arms, mild to moderate tenderness with guarding, and increasing abdominal girth. Hypotension, tachycardia, tachypnea, and cool, clammy skin indicate

that the patient is in hypovolemic shock. You may find that the patient's history includes smoking or cardiovascular disease.

Mesenteric artery ischemia. In this disorder, abdominal rigidity accompanies severe tenderness in the periumbilical region. These symptoms usually develop after 2 to 3 days of persistent, severe, diffuse colicky pain; vomiting; anorexia; diarrhea alternating with constipation; and fever. Hypotension, tachycardia, tachypnea, and cool, clammy skin indicate hypovolemic or septic shock. The patient's history may include a recent episode of hypoperfusion, which may result from one of the following: congestive heart failure, dysrhythmias, or hypotension.

Pancreatitis. A patient with this disorder has abdominal rigidity accompanied by continuous, fulminating pain in the upper abdomen. The pain may radiate to both flanks and the back. To relieve his pain, the patient may bend over, draw his knees to his chest, or move about restlessly.

Other signs and symptoms may include abdominal tenderness or distention, rebound tenderness, hypoactive bowel sounds, nausea, vomiting, fever, pallor, and tachycardia. Turner's or Cullen's sign may indicate hemorrhagic pancreatitis. The patient's history may include alcohol abuse, use of drugs that cause pancreatitis, gallbladder disease, diabetes mellitus, trauma, or a scorpion bite.

Peritonitis. Abdominal rigidity — like the sudden, severe pain that accompanies it — may be localized or generalized in this disorder. If, for example, an inflamed appendix causes local peritonitis, rigidity may be localized in the right lower quadrant. If, however, a perforated ulcer causes widespread peritonitis, rigidity may be generalized. In severe cases, such generalized rigidity may be boardlike.

Associated signs and symptoms include abdominal tenderness and distention, guarding, rebound tenderness, hypoactive or absent bowel sounds, nausea, vomiting, fever, chills, and hyperalgesia. Hypotension, tachycardia, tachypnea, and cool, clammy skin indicate shock associated with septicemia. The patient's history may include a recent episode of fever, flulike symptoms, diarrhea or constipation, abdominal trauma, or peptic ulcer disease.

Other causes
Abdominal rigidity also results from conditions that may not require immediate intervention. These include cholecystitis, diverticulitis, and poisoning by insect bites.

Anuria

A daily urine output of less than 75 ml, anuria occurs infrequently. Why? First, even when renal function is impaired, the kidneys can usually produce 75 ml in 24 hours. Second, because detecting a drop in urine output is relatively simple, disorders that would eventually cause anuria are usually identified and treated before this danger sign develops.

However, when these disorders aren't identified early, anuria can occur, followed rapidly by uremia and other complications of urine retention.

History questions
Explore the patient's problem by asking appropriate questions from this section.
• When did the patient's urine output start to drop — within the last 48 hours or over the last week? How much fluid did he take in during that time?
• Ask if he has any pain. If so, where is it? Is it generalized or localized? Does it radiate?
• Determine if his voiding patterns have changed recently. For instance, has the volume, flow, or frequency been different? Has he experienced dribbling, nocturia, or hematuria? Has he had diarrhea, fever, or chills? What about nausea, vomiting, or hematemesis?
• Does he have an indwelling urinary catheter?
• Find out if he's had recent abdominal, pelvic, renal, or urinary tract surgery.
• Does the patient have a history of kidney disease, urinary tract infection or obstruction, prostate enlargement, renal calculi, neurogenic bladder, congenital anomalies, or other disorders that may result in acute renal failure? (For more information, see *Major causes of acute renal failure,* page 16.) Does he have a history of a cardiac disease that may decrease cardiac output?
• Has he recently taken any drugs that may cause nephrotoxicity, such as amphotericin B, paromomycin, or any of the aminoglycosides or sulfonamides? Determine if he has recently taken drugs that may result in urinary tract calculi or obstructive uropathy, such as acetazolamide, methysergide, or vitamin D. Also determine if he's undergone recent diagnostic tests that use radioiodinated contrast media or received anesthetic agents,

Major causes of acute renal failure

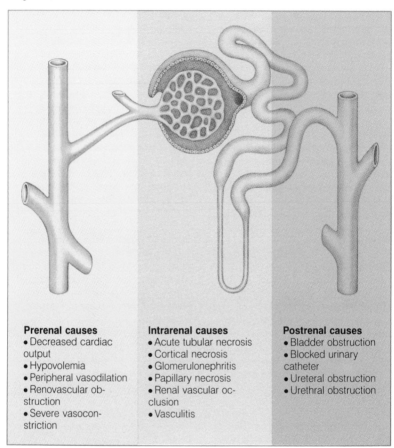

Prerenal causes
- Decreased cardiac output
- Hypovolemia
- Peripheral vasodilation
- Renovascular obstruction
- Severe vasoconstriction

Intrarenal causes
- Acute tubular necrosis
- Cortical necrosis
- Glomerulonephritis
- Papillary necrosis
- Renal vascular occlusion
- Vasculitis

Postrenal causes
- Bladder obstruction
- Blocked urinary catheter
- Ureteral obstruction
- Urethral obstruction

such as methoxyflurane; these drugs can cause nephrotoxicity.

Physical examination

Base your assessment of the patient on the health history information you've collected. Assess his abdomen, making sure you auscultate before palpating and percussing. Using this alternative sequence ensures that you don't affect the frequency or intensity of bowel sounds before you assess them.

Inspection. Observe for abdominal asymmetry, distention, or bulging. Then roll the patient onto his abdomen and note any edema or erythema in the flanks. Cullen's or Turner's sign may indicate renal trauma. Inspect the skin for pallor, decreased turgor, purpura, ecchymoses, uremic crystals, and signs of dehydration. Also, check for fluid retention in the limbs and jugular vein. Inspect the latest urine sample for cloudiness, foul odor, mucus shreds, color changes, or hematuria. If the patient has an indwelling urinary catheter, make sure it's not obstructed or kinked. You may have to irrigate it with normal saline solution to dislodge any obstructions that aren't visible.

Observe his respiratory rate and depth. Does he have difficulty breathing or an abnormal respiratory pattern?

Auscultation. Using the bell of your stethoscope, auscultate over the renal arteries for bruits. Then, with the diaphragm of the stethoscope, auscultate the abdominal quadrants for bowel sounds and note areas of hypoactivity and hyperactivity. Also, auscultate for abnormal breath sounds over the central and peripheral lung fields. Monitor the patient's blood pressure and pulse pressure.

Palpation. Next, palpate the abdominal quadrants, noting any bladder distention or pain, particularly at the costovertebral angle (CVA). Be sure to palpate for renal enlargement or displacement and hepatomegaly. Check peripheral pulses for rate, rhythm, and intensity.

Percussion. Lightly percuss the bladder for fullness and distention. Also, percuss for kidney pain at the CVA.

Life-threatening causes
Your assessment may lead you to suspect one or more of the following.

Acute renal failure. Depending on the underlying cause of renal failure, anuria may develop suddenly or gradually and be accompanied by various other signs and symptoms. In cortical necrosis, for example, anuria develops suddenly and may be preceded by oliguria and accompanied by gross hematuria, flank pain, and fever. In renal artery occlusion, anuria or severe oliguria is accompanied by continuous abdominal and flank pain, nausea, vomiting, decreased bowel sounds, and a fever as high as 102°F (39°C). A patient with anuria usually has a preexisiting condition that's causing acute renal failure, but he may not be aware of it. The patient with acute renal failure may be taking a medication or have received an anesthetic that causes nephrotoxicity.

Urinary tract obstruction. This disorder may cause acute and sometimes complete anuria. Painful or burning urination may precede or alternate with this danger sign. The patient may also experience overflow incontinence or dribbling, increased urinary frequency and nocturia, and decreased or altered urine flow.

Other signs and symptoms include bladder distention, pain and a sensation of fullness in the lower abdomen and groin, severe upper abdominal and flank pain, nausea, and vomiting. You may also note signs of a secondary infection, such as fever, chills, malaise, and cloudy, foul-smelling urine. The patient's diet or medication regimen may predispose him to urinary tract calculi.

Other causes
Anuria also results from conditions that may not require immediate intervention. For instance, when a hypotensive patient's mean blood pressure is 60 mm Hg or lower, anuria results from poor renal perfusion. A congenital anomaly of the urinary tract may also cause anuria.

Apnea

The cessation of spontaneous respiration for longer than 10 seconds, apnea results from one or more of six pathophysiologic mechanisms. Most commonly, it's caused by the progression of a known disorder. But it may develop suddenly and unexpectedly, as with a foreign body airway obstruction. (For more information, see *Identifying causes of apnea*, pages 21 and 22.)

Occasionally, apnea is temporary and self-limiting. More often, though, it requires immediate intervention to save the patient's life. (See *When someone stops breathing*.)

History questions
While resuscitating, explore the patient's problem by asking appropriate questions from this section. Question a family member, a friend, or someone who saw him become apneic.
• Did the apnea begin suddenly or gradually? Did anything happen to the patient right before he became apneic?
• Does the patient have an illness that would predispose him to respiratory failure, such as septic shock, a recent myocardial infarction, or pulmonary embolism?
• Does he have a history of trauma, progressive neuromuscular disease, cardiac disease, or chronic obstructive pulmonary disease?
• Find out if he's taking any medications. Does he have any allergies?

Physical examination
After successful resuscitation, base your assessment of the patient on the health history information you've collected.

Inspection. Observe the rate and depth of the patient's respirations. Does he have difficulty breathing or an abnormal respiratory pattern? Inspect his chest for accessory muscle use, asymmetrical movement of the chest wall during breathing, and labored or paradoxical respirations.

Observe his head, face, neck, and trunk for soft tissue injury, hemorrhage, or skeletal deformity. Note oral or nasal secretions — signs of fluid-filled airways or alveoli. Facial soot and singed nasal hair would indicate a thermal injury to the tracheobronchial tree. Check too for cyanosis, pallor, jugular vein distention, and edema.

If appropriate, perform a neurologic check, evaluating the patient's level of consciousness, orientation, and mental status. Also, test his cranial nerve function, motor function, and sensation. Then evaluate his reflexes in each limb.

Palpation. Gently palpate the chest wall for crepitus associated with fractures of the ribs or sternum. If possible, palpate the posterior chest wall for fractures. Check peripheral pulses for rate, rhythm, and intensity.

Percussion. As you percuss lung fields, listen for increased dullness and hyperresonance.

Auscultation. Listen over each lung lobe for adventitious breath sounds, particularly crackles and rhonchi. If the patient is apneic, you won't hear breath sounds. Also, auscultate the heart for murmurs, pericardial friction rubs, and irregular rhythms. Monitor his blood pressure and pulse pressure.

EMERGENCY INTERVENTION

When someone stops breathing

If someone appears apneic, quickly assess his ABCs—airway, breathing, and circulation.

Airway check
Check for an obstruction and determine if the victim is conscious. If you suspect an obstruction, move him into a supine position and open his airway, using the head-tilt/chin-lift technique.

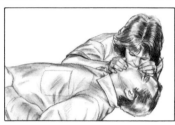

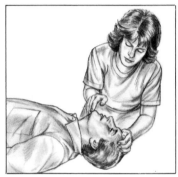

Caution: Use the jaw-thrust technique if you suspect a head or neck injury.

Breathing check
Look, listen, and feel for spontaneous breathing.

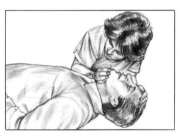

If the victim has stopped breathing, begin giving artificial ventilations, as shown at the top of the next column. As you do, note whether the chest rises. If it doesn't, repeat the head-tilt/

chin-lift technique. If this doesn't work, give abdominal thrusts or use the jaw-thrust lift. In an unconscious patient, you may need to pull down his lower lip and sweep his mouth with two fingers to remove a foreign object. Continue giving artificial ventilations until the victim starts breathing on his own or you begin mechanical ventilation.

Circulation check
Because apnea may result from cardiac arrest (or may cause it), be sure to assess the victim's circulation. Immediately after you establish a patent airway, palpate for the carotid pulse.

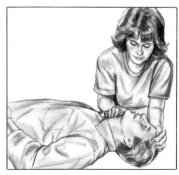

If the victim is a child, palpate the brachial pulse. If you can't feel a pulse, begin giving cardiac compressions.

Life-threatening causes

Your assessment may lead you to suspect one or more of the following.

Airway obstruction. Sudden apnea may result from an obstruction or compression of the trachea or of central or smaller airways. The obstruction blocks airflow, resulting in acute respiratory failure. You won't be able to auscultate breath sounds or feel any air moving through the nose or mouth. The patient may have aspirated vomitus. Or, if he's a trauma victim, he may have aspirated bone, teeth, or blood. An airway obstruction may also occur after exposure to an allergen, or it may result from copious secretions.

Alveolar gas diffusion impairment. An occlusion in the alveolocapillary membrane or fluid in the alveoli may interfere with pulmonary gas exchange, producing apnea. It may arise suddenly — as in near-drowning and pulmonary edema. Or it may develop gradually — as in emphysema. Crackles, labored breathing, and accessory muscle use may precede apnea. The patient's history may include a near-drowning episode or a disorder that causes copious secretions.

Brain stem dysfunction. In this disorder, the brain stem's ability to initiate respirations is destroyed, producing apnea. Apnea may occur suddenly — after trauma, hemorrhage, or infarction — or it may develop gradually, when caused by a degenerative disease or a tumor. Apnea may be preceded by a decreased level of consciousness and motor and sensory deficits. The patient's history may include trauma, progressive neuromuscular disease, or hypertension.

Pleural pressure gradient disruption. A chest wall injury, such as flail chest, may convert pleural pressure from negative to positive, resulting in a collapsed lung and respiratory distress. If the problem isn't treated, apnea may occur. Associated signs include an asymmetrical chest wall and asymmetrical or paradoxical respirations. The patient's history may include chest wall trauma or chronic obstructive pulmonary disease.

Pulmonary capillary perfusion decrease. Apnea may be caused by obstructed pulmonary circulation, most commonly from heart failure or lack of circulatory patency. The danger sign may occur suddenly from cardiac arrest, massive pulmonary embolism, or severe shock. Or it may develop progressively after septic shock or pulmonary hypertension. You may note hypotension, tachycardia, and edema.

Respiratory muscle failure. Trauma or disease that disrupts the mechanics of respiration may result in sudden or gradual apnea. Associated findings may include diaphragmatic or intercostal muscle paralysis from an injury, or respiratory weakness or paralysis associated with an acute or degenerative disease.

Other causes

Episodic or brief apnea also results from certain disorders and drugs and may not require immediate intervention. Prolonged apnea, of course, requires prompt treatment.

Disorders. In sleep apnea, spontaneous breathing stops temporarily; it's usually associated with snoring, insomnia, and daytime fatigue. Premature infants may develop

PATHOPHYSIOLOGY

Identifying causes of apnea

This list itemizes the six pathophysiologic mechanisms that cause apnea along with conditions that trigger them.

Airway obstruction
- Airway edema
- Airway occlusion by tongue
- Airway occlusion by tumor
- Anaphylaxis
- Asthma
- Bronchospasm
- Chronic bronchitis
- Diffuse atelectasis
- Foreign body aspiration
- Hemothorax or pneumothorax
- Mucus plugs
- Obstructive sleep apnea
- Secretion retention
- Tracheal or bronchial rupture

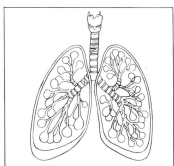

Impaired alveolar gas diffusion
- Adult respiratory distress syndrome
- Diffuse pneumonia
- Emphysema
- Near-drowning
- Pulmonary edema
- Pulmonary fibrosis
- Secretion retention

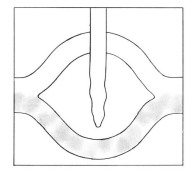

Brain stem dysfunction
- Brain abscess
- Brain tumor
- Cerebral hemorrhage
- Cerebral infarction
- Encephalitis
- Head trauma
- Hypoventilatory sleep apnea
- Increased intracranial pressure
- Meningitis
- Opiates
- Pontine-medullary hemorrhage or infarction
- Transtentorial herniation

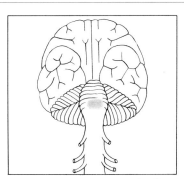

(*continued*)

PATHOPHYSIOLOGY

Identifying causes of apnea *(continued)*

Disruption of pleural pressure gradient
- Flail chest
- Open chest wounds

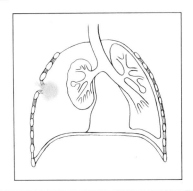

Decreased pulmonary capillary perfusion
- Cardiac arrest
- Dysrhythmias
- Myocardial infarction
- Pulmonary embolism
- Pulmonary hypertension
- Shock

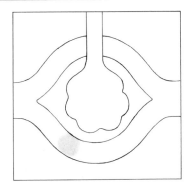

Respiratory muscle failure
- Amyotrophic lateral sclerosis
- Botulism
- Diphtheria
- Guillain-Barré syndrome
- Myasthenia gravis
- Neuromuscular blocking agents
- Pesticide poisoning
- Phrenic nerve paralysis
- Rupture of the diaphragm
- Spinal cord injury

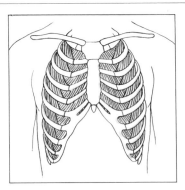

apneic episodes caused by their immature central nervous systems (CNSs).

Drugs. CNS depressants, such as alcohol, anesthetics, barbiturates, and narcotic analgesics, may result in hypoventilation or apnea. A patient may develop respiratory depression or apnea after an I.V. infusion of diazepam or other benzodiazepines, especially when given with other CNS depressants. Elderly and acutely ill patients are especially susceptible to such combinations of drugs. Also, neuro-muscular blocking agents — such as pancuronium and succinylcholine, and anticholinesterase inhibi-tors — may produce respiratory muscle paralysis, causing sudden apnea.

Back pain

This symptom may originate in several areas — the abdominopelvic viscera, the vertebral structures, the spinal cord and its vasculature, and the muscles of the thoracic, lumbar, and sacral regions. But back pain indicates danger only when it's referred from the abdominopelvic viscera. Typically, this pain isn't affected by activity or rest, unlike back pain associated with muscles, vertebral structures, or the spinal cord, which worsens with activity and improves with rest. Frequently, pain from a neoplasm will be relieved by walking and will worsen at night.

History questions
Explore the patient's problem by asking appropriate questions from this section.

- Where is the pain? Is it localized or diffused? Does it radiate? When did it start? Did it begin suddenly or gradually? Is it worse at a certain time of day?
- Ask the patient to describe his pain. Is it sharp or dull, shooting or burning? Find out if it's constant or intermittent. If it's intermittent, how long does it last? Is his pain associated with activity? Does it change with activity, such as walking, coughing, or stretching?
- Find out if the patient has had recent episodes of fever, nausea, vomiting, abdominal tenderness, or abdominal rigidity. Does he feel any unusual sensations in his legs? What about changes in his ability to use his leg muscles? Has he partici-pated in any activities that cause sudden or extreme spinal flexion or rotation? Has he had urinary frequency or urgency or painful urination? Is his urine cloudy or pink?
- Does the patient have a history of trauma; back surgery; urinary tract surgery or procedures, ob-struction, or infections? Does he have diabetes mellitus? Has he ever had a spinal cord injury, a progressive neuromuscular disorder, peptic ulcers, frequent heartburn or epigastric distress, or urinary tract infections? What about smok-ing, routine use of alcohol or drugs, or a family history of cardiovascular disease?
- If the patient is a woman, obtain a menstrual history. Ask specifically about any premenstrual or postmen-strual symptoms.
- Ask the patient if he's taken any drugs that may cause pancreatitis, such as azathioprine, ethacrynic acid, or furosemide. What about opiates, oral contraceptives, sulfona-mides, thiazide diuretics, or cortico-steroids?

Physical examination

Base your assessment of the patient on the health history information you've collected.

Inspection. Observe the rate and depth of the patient's respirations. Does he have difficulty breathing or an abnormal respiratory pattern?

Check the skin for pallor, mottling, diaphoresis, discoloration, and edema (especially of the legs). These signs may indicate decreased oxygenation, venostasis, lowered cardiac output, or shock.

Inspect the back, legs, and abdomen for signs of trauma, such as lacerations, bruises, and erythema. Also look for signs of thrombophlebitis, including redness, swelling, and warmth over the leg veins. Cullen's or Turner's sign may indicate trauma or hemorrhagic pancreatitis.

Then check for abdominal distention. Take a baseline measurement of abdominal girth at the umbilicus. A later increase may indicate bleeding, which can cause back pain. Also inspect the patient's urine for color and odor.

Auscultation. If you suspect that the pain is referred from the abdomen, auscultate before palpating and percussing. Using this alternative sequence ensures that you don't alter the frequency or intensity of bowel sounds before you assess them.

Auscultate each abdominal quadrant for bowel sounds. Be sure to auscultate over the same spot for at least 5 minutes to distinguish between hypoactive or absent bowel sounds. Then auscultate over the abdominal aorta for bruits. Also auscultate over the lungs for crackles, which may indicate congestive heart failure (CHF).

Monitor blood pressure and pulse pressure.

Palpation. Next, palpate the abdomen and epigastric and pelvic areas for enlarged organs, masses, abdominal rigidity, and tenderness. If you palpate a mass, note whether it's pulsating. If it is, don't palpate deeply. Check peripheral pulses for rate, rhythm, and intensity, being careful to note if the pedal and femoral pulses are weak or absent in one or both legs.

Gently palpate the painful area for excessive muscle tone, contraction, or spasm. Also palpate over the kidneys — especially over the costovertebral angle (CVA) — to see if the pain increases. Check for pain or tenderness in the paravertebral muscles.

Percussion. As you gently percuss each abdominal quadrant, note any increased pain, tenderness, or abnormal sounds. Using a reflex hammer, test the Achilles and patellar reflexes and note any abnormal responses.

Life-threatening causes

Your assessment may lead you to suspect one or more of the following.

Abdominal aortic aneurysm (dissecting). Low back pain and dull upper abdominal pain often accompany a rapidly enlarging aneurysm and may indicate the early stages of a rupture. The patient feels more pain when lying down and less when sitting up or leaning forward. You may palpate tenderness over the area of the aneurysm and a pulsating epigastric mass, which stops pulsating after the rupture. You may auscultate a systolic bruit.

Other signs and symptoms include mottled skin below the waist, absent femoral and pedal pulses, blood pressure lower in the legs than the arms, mild to moderate abdominal tenderness with guarding, and abdominal rigidity. Hypotension, tachycardia, tachypnea, and cool, clammy skin indicate hypovolemic shock. The history may include smoking or cardiovascular disease.

Appendicitis. A patient will have vague, dull back pain radiating from the epigastric or umbilical region accompanied by dull abdominal discomfort or severe abdominal pain. Typically, the pain follows anorexia, nausea, vomiting, diarrhea, or constipation. The patient may experience milder or flulike symptoms for a few hours to a few days before seeking medical attention. Or the onset may be sudden. The pain becomes localized at McBurney's point and may be accompanied by abdominal rigidity, increasing tenderness (especially over McBurney's point), rebound tenderness, and retractions on respiration.

Pancreatitis. Fulminating, continuous abdominal pain that may radiate to the back and both flanks characterizes this disorder. For relief, a patient may bend over, draw his knees to his chest, or move about restlessly. Abdominal tenderness, nausea, vomiting, fever, pallor, or tachycardia may also occur. Some patients may also have abdominal rigidity and distention, rebound tenderness, and hypoactive bowel sounds. Cullen's or Turner's sign may indicate hemorrhagic pancreatitis. The patient's history may include alcohol abuse, use of drugs that produce pancreatitis (thiazide diuretics, for instance), gallbladder disease, diabetes mellitus, trauma, or a scorpion bite.

Perforated ulcer. In this disorder, sudden, severe, prostrating epigastric pain radiates to the back. You may note boardlike abdominal rigidity, abdominal tenderness with guarding, generalized rebound tenderness, absent bowel sounds, fever, tachycardia, hypotension, and grunting, shallow breaths. The patient's history may include gastric or duodenal ulcer, frequent stomach upset, heartburn, or epigastric pain associated with bloody stool.

Pyelonephritis (acute). The patient will have progressive back pain or tenderness in the flank area accompanied by CVA and abdominal pain in one or both lower quadrants. This pain may radiate to the groin. Associated signs and symptoms include high fever, shaking chills, nausea, vomiting, dysuria, hematuria, nocturia, and urinary frequency and urgency.

The patient may have recently undergone a urinary tract procedure. Also, his history may include an infection (especially of the urinary tract), a urinary tract obstruction, neurogenic bladder, compromised renal function, or diabetes mellitus. Sexually active or pregnant women are susceptible to this disorder.

Renal vein occlusion. When thrombosis has a rapid onset, the patient may feel severe lumbar pain accompanied by CVA and epigastric tenderness. You may also note fever, pallor, hematuria, proteinuria, and peripheral edema. In bilateral obstruction, your examination will reveal enlarged kidneys, oliguria, and other signs of uremia. The patient may also be hypertensive. His history may include thrombophlebitis of the inferior vena cava or the lower legs, CHF, or periarteritis.

Other causes
Back pain can result from certain disorders that may not require immediate intervention. It can also result from procedures.

Disorders. Intervertebral disk rupture, lumbosacral or sacroiliac sprain, spinal stenosis, spondylolisthesis, transverse process fracture, vertebral compression, vertebral osteomyelitis, and vertebral osteoporosis may cause back pain. So may premenstrual syndrome, dysmenorrhea, endometriosis, postural imbalance associated with pregnancy, cholecystitis, myeloma, prostatic cancer, benign spinal neoplasm, Reiter's syndrome, renal calculi, and sickle cell crisis.

Procedures. Diagnostic procedures, such as lumbar puncture and myelography, may produce temporary back pain.

Bowel sounds, absent

Bowel sounds are considered absent when you can't hear them after auscultating for 5 minutes in each abdominal quadrant.

The silence results from a cessation of peristalsis, caused by mechanical or vascular obstruction or neurogenic inhibition. When peristalsis stops, gas from bowel contents and fluid from the bowel wall accumulate, distending the lumen.

History questions
Explore the patient's problem by asking appropriate questions from this section.
● Does the patient have abdominal pain? If so, when did it begin?

Has it gotten worse? Where is it? Does it radiate?
● Ask if the patient feels bloated or has been passing flatus. Find out when he had his last bowel movement. An absence of bowel movements could indicate complete obstruction and paralytic ileus. Determine if he's had diarrhea or passed pencil-thin stools — possible signs of a developing luminal obstruction.
● Did the patient have an accident that could have caused vascular clots? Even a seemingly minor accident — falling off a stepladder, for instance — could produce this effect.
● Determine if he's had recent abdominal surgery, which could lead to paralytic ileus. Has he had a recent episode of hypoperfusion, which may result from congestive heart failure, cardiac dysrhythmias, or hypotension?
● Has the patient ever had an abdominal tumor, hernia, or adhesions from surgery? What about radiation therapy of the abdomen or pelvis? Is there a history of acute pancreatitis, diverticulitis, or gynecologic infection that may have led to intra-abdominal infection and bowel dysfunction? Has the patient ever had a toxic condition, such as uremia? Does he have a spinal cord injury?
● What medications is the patient taking?

Physical examination
Base your assessment of the patient on the health history information you've collected. Assess the abdomen, making sure you auscultate before palpating and percussing. Using this alternative sequence ensures that you don't affect the frequency or intensity of bowel sounds before you assess them.

Inspection. Check for abdominal distention. Then take a baseline measurement of the patient's abdominal girth at the umbilicus. An increase may indicate bleeding.

Observe the rate and depth of his respirations. See if he's having difficulty breathing or if he has an abnormal respiratory pattern.

Auscultation. Using the diaphragm of your stethoscope, auscultate the abdominal quadrants for bowel sounds. To distinguish between absent sounds and hypoactive ones, make sure you listen in the same spot for at least 5 minutes (see *Are bowel sounds really absent?*). Then with the bell of the stethoscope, auscultate over the abdominal aorta for abdominal bruits. Monitor the patient's blood pressure and pulse pressure.

Palpation. As you palpate each quadrant, note any abdominal masses. Also, check for abdominal rigidity and guarding, which may indicate peritoneal irritation. Be sure your hands are warm when you assess for abdominal rigidity. If they're cold, your touch may make the abdominal muscles contract. Then check peripheral pulses for rate, rhythm, and intensity.

Percussion. Gently percuss the abdomen. You'll hear dull percussion sounds over fluid-filled areas and tympanic sounds over pockets of gas.

Life-threatening causes

Your assessment may lead you to suspect one or more of the following.

Complete mechanical intestinal obstruction. Absent bowel sounds follow a period of hyperactive bowel sounds in this disorder. The silent

Are bowel sounds really absent?

Before concluding that your patient's bowel sounds are absent, ask yourself these three questions:

Did you use the diaphragm of your stethoscope to auscultate for the bowel sounds?
The diaphragm detects high-frequency sounds, such as bowel sounds, whereas the bell detects low-frequency sounds, such as vascular bruits or venous hums.

Did you listen in the same spot for at least 5 minutes?
Normally, bowel sounds occur every 5 to 15 seconds, but a single bowel sound may last less than a second.

Did you listen for bowel sounds in all quadrants?
Bowel sounds may be absent in one abdominal quadrant, but present in another.

abdomen is accompanied by acute, colicky pain in the quadrant of the obstruction. Pain may also radiate to the flank or lumbar region. Associated signs and symptoms include abdominal distention and bloating, constipation, nausea, and vomiting. The higher the blockage, the earlier and more severe the vomiting. In some cases, you may palpate an abdominal mass. During the late stages, fever, rebound tenderness, and abdominal rigidity develop. Tachycardia, tachypnea, hypotension, and cool, clammy skin indicate shock associated with dehydration and hypovolemia. The patient's history may include episodes of bloody stools, internal or external hernias, and abdominal or pelvic radiation

Intestinal obstruction: Recognizing the complications

A patient's intestinal obstruction may result from either mechanical or non-mechanical causes. Mechanical causes include tumors, adhesions and fecal impaction; nonmechanical causes include paralytic ileus caused by abdominal surgery, retroperitoneal hemorrhage, and mesenteric artery ischemia.

Both can lead to shock, making quick intervention vital. The flowchart below traces the path of complications that can result from intestinal obstruction.

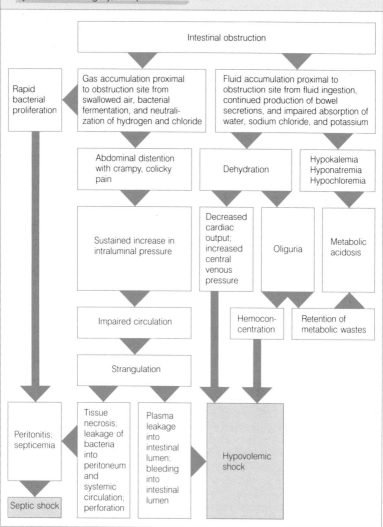

Intestinal obstruction

Rapid bacterial proliferation

Gas accumulation proximal to obstruction site from swallowed air, bacterial fermentation, and neutralization of hydrogen and chloride

Fluid accumulation proximal to obstruction site from fluid ingestion, continued production of bowel secretions, and impaired absorption of water, sodium chloride, and potassium

Abdominal distention with crampy, colicky pain

Dehydration

Hypokalemia
Hyponatremia
Hypochloremia

Sustained increase in intraluminal pressure

Decreased cardiac output; increased central venous pressure

Oliguria

Metabolic acidosis

Impaired circulation

Hemoconcentration

Retention of metabolic wastes

Strangulation

Peritonitis; septicemia

Septic shock

Tissue necrosis; leakage of bacteria into peritoneum and systemic circulation; perforation

Plasma leakage into intestinal lumen; bleeding into intestinal lumen

Hypovolemic shock

therapy or surgery that caused adhesions. (See *Intestinal obstruction: Recognizing the complications.*)

Mesenteric artery infarction. In this disorder, bowel sounds cease after a brief period of hyperactive sounds. Sudden, colicky, severe midepigastric or periumbilical pain develops, then becomes more severe and generalized. Abdominal distention, copious vomiting, bloody diarrhea, constipation, fever, and possibly bruits are also present. Fever above 102° F (39° C), abdominal rigidity, and other signs of peritonitis indicate necrosis. The patient's history may include an episode of hypoperfusion, possibly associated with congestive heart failure, cardiac dysrhythmias, or hypotension.

Paralytic (adynamic) ileus. The cardinal sign of this disorder is absent bowel sounds. Associated signs and symptoms include abdominal distention, generalized discomfort, tympany, and obstipation or passage of flatus and small, liquid stools. If the disorder follows acute abdominal infection, the patient may also have a fever and abdominal pain. His history may include recent abdominal surgery or any peritoneal insult. The disorder may develop with a spinal, pelvic, or rib fracture; trauma; retroperitoneal hemorrhage; pyelonephritis; ureteral calculi; pneumonia; myocardial infarction; sepsis; and metabolic abnormalities.

Perforated ulcer. A patient with this disorder may have absent bowel sounds accompanied by sudden, severe, prostrating epigastric pain that radiates to his back. You may also note boardlike abdominal rigidity; tenderness with guarding; generalized rebound tenderness; grunting, shallow

respirations; and fever. Tachycardia, tachypnea, hypotension, and cool, clammy skin indicate hypovolemic shock. The patient's history may include a known gastric or duodenal ulcer or complaints of frequent stomach upset, heartburn, or epigastric pain.

Other cause
Bowel sounds are normally absent after abdominal surgery — the result of anesthetics and surgical manipulation.

Bowel sounds, hyperactive

Increased intestinal motility (or peristalsis) produces hyperactive bowel sounds, typically described as loud, rapid, rushing, gurgling, or tinkling waves of sounds. Usually, you'll need to use the diaphragm of your stethoscope to hear bowel sounds. However, certain bowel sounds known as borborygmi are loud enough to be heard without a stethoscope.

Hyperactive bowel sounds may alternate with periods of silence, so be sure you auscultate long enough to detect this pattern.

History questions
Explore the patient's problem by asking appropriate questions from this section.
• Is the patient also having abdominal pain? If so, how does the onset of pain correspond to the hyperactive sounds? Has he been vomiting, or is he experiencing constipation or diarrhea? If he's been vomiting, was the vomitus bloody? Is he having or has he had bloody stools?

Distinguishing among types of bowel sounds

> The sounds of air and fluid moving through the GI tract are known as bowel sounds. These sounds usually occur every 5 to 15 seconds, but their frequency may be irregular. For example, bowel sounds are normally more active just before and after a meal. Their duration may vary from less than a second to several seconds.
>
> These descriptions should help you to distinguish among the types of bowel sounds:
>
> • *Normal bowel sounds* are usually described as murmuring, gurgling, or tinkling.
> • *Hyperactive bowel sounds* can be characterized as loud, gurgling, splashing, and rushing. They're higher-pitched and, of course, occur more frequently than normal sounds.
> • *Hypoactive bowel sounds* can be described as softer and lower-pitched than normal sounds. They also occur less frequently.

Ask if he's experienced weakness, extreme tiredness, fainting, or palpitations.
• Ask too about recent eruptions of gastroenteritis among family members, friends, or co-workers. If the patient has traveled recently, even within the United States, ask whether he's aware of any endemic illnesses in the regions he visited. Does the patient have known food allergies or has he recently ingested any unusual foods or fluids?
• Determine if there's a history of abdominal tumors, hernias, or adhesions from surgery or radiation therapy of the abdomen or pelvis. Does the patient have a history of GI disorders—inflammatory bowel disease or peptic ulcer

disease, for instance? Has he ever had an episode of severe trauma, severe illness, burns, central nervous system (CNS) trauma or operations, sepsis, or other severe infections that could predispose him to stress ulcers?
• Is the patient taking or does he routinely take drugs that can cause GI bleeding? These drugs include salicylates, steroids, nonsteroidal anti-inflammatory agents, potassium supplements, and antineoplastics.

Physical examination
Base your assessment of the patient on the health history you've taken. Assess his abdomen, making sure you auscultate before palpating and percussing. Using this alternative sequence ensures that you don't affect the frequency and intensity of bowel sounds before you auscultate them.

Inspection. Peristaltic waves may be visible in very thin patients, so observe for them, if appropriate. Then inspect the patient for abdominal distention. Take a baseline measurement of his abdominal girth at the umbilicus. An increase may indicate bleeding.
Observe the rate and depth of his respirations. Does he have difficulty breathing or an abnormal respiratory rate?

Auscultation. With the diaphragm of the stethoscope, auscultate the abdominal quadrants, listening long enough to determine if periods of silence alternate with periods of hyperactivity. (For more information, see *Distinguishing among types of bowel sounds.*) Also monitor his blood pressure and pulse pressure.

Palpation. As you palpate all quadrants, check for abdominal masses. Feel for epigastric tenderness and abdominal rigidity, which may indicate peritoneal irritation. Remember, your hands should be warm when you assess for abdominal rigidity. If they're cold, your touch may make the abdominal muscles contract. Then check his peripheral pulses, noting rate, rhythm, and intensity.

Percussion. Gently percuss the patient's abdomen. You'll hear dull percussion sounds over fluid-filled areas and tympanic sounds over pockets of gas.

Life-threatening causes
Your assessment may lead you to suspect one or more of the following.

GI hemorrhage. Hyperactive bowel sounds give you the most immediate indication of persistent GI bleeding. Associated signs and symptoms may include abdominal distention, hematemesis, bloody diarrhea, rectal passage of bright red blood clots and jellylike material, and abdominal pain. The patient may have recently experienced weakness, malaise, dyspnea, palpitations, faintness, sweating, or syncope. Hypotension, tachycardia, tachypnea, and cool, clammy skin indicate hypovolemic shock. His history may include GI ulcers, use of drugs that cause GI bleeding, severe trauma, severe illness, burns, CNS trauma or operations, sepsis, or severe infections that cause stress ulcers.

Mechanical intestinal obstruction. High-pitched, tinkling, hyperactive bowel sounds are accompanied by brief episodes of intense, colicky abdominal pain that occur every few minutes. Other signs and symptoms include tympany, abdominal disten-tion, guarding and tenderness, and visible peristaltic waves. Distal to the obstruction, you may note lower-pitched hypoactive or absent sounds. Obstipation and pain-induced agitation also occur. In jejunal and duodenal obstruction, nausea and bilious vomiting develop early. Often, in distal small-bowel or large-bowel obstruction, nausea and vomiting are feculent. Complete bowel obstruction causes absent bowel sounds. Hypotension, tachycardia, tachypnea, and cool, clammy skin indicate hypovolemic shock. The patient's history may include bloody stools or previous abdominal radiation therapy or abdominal surgery that may cause adhesions.

Other causes
Certain causes of hyperactive bowel sounds may not require immediate intervention.

Activities of daily living. Erratic eating habits and excessive ingestion of certain foods, such as unripened fruit, may bring on hyperactive bowel sounds.

Disorders. Crohn's disease, food hypersensitivity, gastroenteritis, and acute ulcerative colitis can cause hyperactive bowel sounds.

Bowel sounds, hypoactive

Detected by auscultating with the diaphragm of the stethoscope, hypoactive bowel sounds result from diminished peristalsis. These sounds occur less frequently than normal bowel sounds; they're also lower-pitched and not as loud.

Hypoactive bowel sounds don't always indicate an emergency.

During sleep, for instance, they're considered normal. But hypoactive bowels sounds are an early sign of some life-threatening disorders.

History questions

Explore the patient's problem by asking appropriate questions from this section.

• Is the patient in pain? If so, when did the pain begin? Has it gotten worse? Where exactly is the pain? Is it localized or generalized? Or does it radiate to another area?

• Ask if the patient has been vomiting. If so, find out when it started, how often it occurs, and whether the vomitus looks bloody.

• Have the patient's bowel habits changed recently? Note if he's been constipated. Ask when he last had a bowel movement or expelled flatus. Has he had diarrhea or passed pencil-thin stools — possible signs of a developing luminal obstruction? An absence of bowel movements may indicate a complete obstruction or paralytic ileus.

• Did the patient have an accident that could have caused vascular clots? Even a seemingly minor accident, such as falling off a stepladder, could produce this effect.

• Has the patient ever had a condition that could cause an obstruction — an abdominal tumor or hernia, for example. What about abdominal or pelvic surgery or radiation therapy that may cause obstruction or adhesions? Has the patient had a condition that could cause paralytic ileus, such as pancreatitis; a bowel inflammation or a gynecologic infection, which may produce peritonitis; a toxic condition, such as uremia; severe pain; or a spinal cord injury? Recent abdominal surgery may also cause paralytic ileus.

• Is the patient taking any drugs that decrease peristalsis, such as opiates, anticholinergics, phenothiazines, tricyclic antidepressants, or vinca alkaloids?

Physical examination

Base your assessment of the patient on the health history information you've collected. Assess his abdomen, making sure you auscultate before palpating and percussing. Using this alternative sequence ensures that you don't affect the frequency and intensity of bowel sounds before you auscultate them.

Inspection. Observe the abdomen for distention and note any surgical scars or obvious masses. Then take a baseline measurement of the patient's abdominal girth at the umbilicus. An increase may indicate bleeding.

Observe his rate and depth of respiration. See if he has difficulty breathing or an abnormal respiratory pattern.

Auscultation. Use the diaphragm of the stethoscope to auscultate the abdominal quadrants for bowel sounds. To distinguish between hypoactive sounds and absent sounds, auscultate for at least 5 minutes in the same spot. Then with the bell of the stethoscope, auscultate over the abdominal aorta to detect any abdominal bruits. Monitor the patient's blood pressure and pulse pressure.

Palpation. Check all quadrants for abdominal masses. Also, palpate for abdominal rigidity and guarding — indications of peritoneal irritation. Make sure your hands are warm when you assess for abdominal rigidity. If they're cold, the patient's abdominal muscles may contract under your touch. Then check the rate, rhythm, and intensity of peripheral pulses.

Percussion. Next, gently percuss the abdomen. Dull percussion sounds indicate fluid-filled areas; tympanic sounds, pockets of gas.

Life-threatening causes

Your assessment may lead you to suspect one or more of the following.

Mechanical intestinal obstruction. In this disorder, hypoactive bowel sounds follow a period of hyperactive bowel sounds. The patient may also have acute, colicky abdominal pain in the quadrant of obstruction, possibly radiating to the flank or lumbar regions.

Associated signs and symptoms include abdominal distention and bloating, constipation, nausea, and vomiting. The higher the blockage, the earlier and more severe the vomiting. You may palpate an abdominal mass. In the late stages, the patient may have a fever, rebound tenderness, and abdominal rigidity. Tachycardia, tachypnea, hypotension, and cool, clammy skin indicate shock associated with dehydration and hypovolemia. The patient's history may include episodes of bloody stools, internal or external hernias, and abdominal or pelvic radiation therapy or surgery that caused adhesions.

Mesenteric artery infarction. After a brief period of hyperactivity, bowel sounds become hypoactive then quickly stop. The patient feels sudden, colicky, severe midepigastric or periumbilical pain, which becomes more severe and generalized as the infarction progresses.

Other possible signs and symptoms include abdominal distention, copious vomiting, bloody diarrhea, constipation, fever, and bruits. Fever above 102° F (39° C), abdominal rigidity, and other signs of peritonitis signify necrosis. The patient's history may include an episode of hypoperfusion, possibly associated with congestive heart failure, cardiac dysrhythmias, or hypotension.

Paralytic (adynamic) ileus. The cardinal sign of this disorder is hypoactive bowel sounds that may stop. Associated signs and symptoms include abdominal distention, generalized discomfort, tympany, and obstipation or flatus with small, liquid stools. If the disorder follows an acute abdominal infection, the patient may also have a fever and abdominal pain. His history may include recent abdominal surgery or any peritoneal insult. Paralytic ileus may also develop with a spinal, pelvic, or rib fracture; trauma; retroperitoneal hemorrhage; pyelonephritis; ureteral calculi; pneumonia; myocardial infarction; sepsis; or metabolic abnormalities.

Pancreatitis. Hypoactive bowel sounds often accompany the cardinal signs of acute pancreatitis — abdominal rigidity and fulminating continuous upper abdominal pain that may radiate to the flanks and back. To relieve the pain, the patient may bend forward, draw his knees to his chest, or move about restlessly. Other signs and symptoms include abdominal distention, abdominal tenderness, rebound tenderness, nausea, vomiting, fever, pallor, and tachycardia. Turner's or Cullen's sign may indicate hemorrhagic pancreatitis. The patient may have a history of alcohol abuse or use of drugs that may cause pancreatitis. His history may also include gallbladder disease, a scorpion bite, diabetes mellitus, or trauma.

Other causes

Hypoactive bowel sounds don't always signal the need for immediate intervention. They can result from daily activities, drugs, and procedures.

Activities of daily living. Bowel distention from swallowing too much air while eating may produce hypoactive bowel sounds.

Drugs. Certain drugs reduce intestinal motility, causing hypoactive bowel sounds. These include opiates, such as codeine; anticholinergics, such as propantheline bromide; phenothiazines, such as chlorpromazine; tricyclic antidepressants, such as amitriptyline; and vinca alkaloids, such as vincristine. General or spinal anesthetics produce transient hypoactive sounds.

Procedures. After radiation therapy or abdominal surgery, a patient may develop hypoactive bowel sounds.

Bradycardia

A heart rate of less than 60 beats/ minute, bradycardia may occur normally in young adults, athletes, and elderly people. It's also a normal response to vagal stimulation triggered by coughing, vomiting, or straining during a bowel movement. In such cases, the heart rate rarely falls below 40 beats/minute. But when bradycardia results from a pathologic cause — a cardiovascular disorder, for example — the heart rate may plummet to 1 beat/minute.

By itself, bradycardia is nonspecific. When accompanied by chest pain, hypotension, dizziness, shortness of breath, or a decreased level of consciousness, it may indicate a life-threatening disorder.

History questions

Explore the patient's problem by asking appropriate questions from this section.

• Does he have chest pain, dyspnea, hypotension, headaches, or palpitations? Is he dizzy or fatigued? Does he feel weak, especially in the legs? What was he doing when the bradycardia began?

• Ask if he's had bradycardia before. If so, what relieved it? Does he have a family history of it?

• Was the patient exposed to cold for a prolonged period? An elderly person with a low income may have inadequate heat in his home. An alcoholic or homeless person may have slept outside in cold weather. Or the patient may have been hiking or camping in cold weather.

• Does he routinely engage in strenuous aerobic activity? If so, what kind and for how long? Has he had a recent episode of head, neck, or spinal cord trauma? Did he recently undergo cardiac catheterization, electrophysiologic studies, cardiac surgery, or suctioning?

• Find out if he has a congenital heart defect, systemic infection, brain tumor, cardiomyopathy, or cirrhosis of the liver. Has he ever had a cerebrovascular accident (CVA) or a cardiac disorder, such as myocardial ischemia, myocardial infarction (MI), or heart block? Does he have a history of endocrine or metabolic disorders?

• Is the patient taking any drugs that slow the heart rate, such as digoxin, pilocarpine, or quinidine? Has he taken a drug that may cause MI, such as dextrothyroxine?

Has he taken a large dose of phenothiazines or drunk a lot of alcohol?

Physical examination
Base your assessment of the patient on the health history information you've collected.

Inspection. Observe the patient's respiratory rate and depth. Does he have difficulty breathing or an abnormal respiratory pattern? Then check his skin for signs of dehydration and temperature changes. Inspect his nail beds and mucous membranes for peripheral and central cyanosis — late signs of inadequate cardiac output.

Look for pupillary changes and assess the patient's level of consciousness. Then check for edema or neck vein distention. To determine if the patient has experienced trauma, look for bruising and lacerations.

Palpation. Next, palpate the radial pulse while auscultating the apical pulse, comparing the pulses for a full minute (see *Bradycardia and pulse deficit: How to tell them apart*). As you palpate the muscles of the arms and legs, note decreased muscle tone or rigidity. Then test the strength of each limb, comparing one side to the other. Also, palpate the upper abdomen for an enlarged liver.

Percussion. To check for abdominal pain or tenderness, lightly percuss the entire abdomen. Also, note any abnormal percussion sounds. Then assess the brachial, patellar, and Achilles tendon reflexes, noting any abnormal response.

Auscultation. Listen to the patient's heart rate and rhythm, and note any

Bradycardia and pulse deficit: How to tell them apart

Sometimes, when you detect a low peripheral pulse rate, the problem isn't bradycardia — it's a pulse deficit. To determine which one is causing the low pulse rate, you need to take the patient's apical-radial pulse. Here's how:

Auscultate the patient's heart rate while palpating his radial pulse. If you hear beats that you can't palpate, the patient has a pulse deficit, not bradycardia. The difference between the number of apical beats and the number of radial beats is the pulse deficit.

abnormal heart sounds. Auscultate each lung field for diminished or absent breath sounds, and adventitious sounds such as crackles. Also monitor the patient's blood pressure and pulse pressure.

Life-threatening causes
Your assessment may lead you to suspect one or more of the following.

Cardiac dysrhythmia. Intermittent or sustained bradycardia usually accompanies hypotension, palpitations, chest pain, dizziness, weakness, and fatigue in this disorder. The patient may be taking digitalis, or he may have a history of cardiac dysrhythmias such as heart block.

Cervical spinal injury. Transient or sustained bradycardia will be associated with sympathetic denervation. The more severe the spinal injury, the longer the bradycardia. Associated signs and symptoms may include hypotension, hypothermia, slowed peristalsis, leg or partial arm paralysis, and respiratory muscle paralysis. The history may include a spinal cord injury or tumor.

Hypothermia. When the body's core temperature drops below 89.6° F (32° C), bradycardia occurs. You may also note hypotension, bradypnea, shivering, peripheral cyanosis, confusion leading to stupor and coma, muscle rigidity, joint stiffness, and cardiac dysrhythmias. The patient has probably been exposed to the cold for a few hours. He may also have ingested a large dose of phenothiazines or a large amount of alcohol. His history may include hypothyroidism, hypoadrenalism, advanced cirrhosis, CVA, or cervical spine injury.

Increased intracranial pressure. Occurring late in this disorder, bradycardia follows hypertension, tachycardia, altered mental status, headache, and perhaps projectile vomiting. The bradycardia will be accompanied by tachypnea or apneustic respirations and a widening pulse pressure. The patient may complain of a persistent headache. You may note progressive loss of consciousness, seizures, and pupillary changes. Cheyne-Stokes respirations indicate deteriorating brain function. His history may include systemic infection, head trauma, brain surgery, brain tumor, or metabolic or cardiac disease.

Myocardial infarction. Mild or severe bradycardia, which results from vagal stimulation or inadequate perfusion of the conduction system, may accompany the cardinal signs of an MI. These include crushing chest pain that may radiate to the jaw, shoulder, arm, or epigastrium; dyspnea; anxiety; nausea or vomiting; diaphoresis; cool, pale, or cyanotic skin; and a feeling of impending doom. The patient may be hypotensive or hypertensive. You may auscultate an atrial gallop, murmur, and, occasionally, an irregular pulse. The patient may have a history or a family history of cardiac disease. He may have recently experienced extreme stress. His life-style may include excessive sodium and fat intake, little or no exercise, and smoking. He may also be taking cocaine, dextrothyroxine, estramustine phosphate sodium, or recombinant interleukin-2, any of which can cause an MI.

Other causes

Bradycardia doesn't always signal the need for immediate intervention. Certain disorders that aren't life-threatening, as well as drugs and procedures, can cause this sign.

Disorders. Bradycardia appears in patients with cardiomyopathy, congenital heart disease, or hypothyroidism. Fetal bradycardia — a heart rate of less than 120 beats/minute — may develop from prolonged labor or complications of delivery, including compression of the umbilicus, partial abruptio placentae, and placenta previa.

Drugs. Transient bradycardia may result from diazepam, I.V. nitroglycerin, protamine sulfate, quinidine, beta-adrenergic blockers, calcium channel blockers, cardiac glycosides, narcotics, sympatholytics, and topical miotics such as pilocarpine.

Procedures. Cardiac catheterization and electrophysiologic studies may induce temporary bradycardia. Suctioning produces hypoxia and vagal stimulation, causing bradycardia. Edema or damage to conduction tissues from cardiac surgery will also trigger bradycardia.

Bradypnea

Bradypnea refers to a pattern of regular respirations at a rate below 12 breaths/minute. Because respiratory rates are higher in children than in adults, pediatric bradypnea is defined according to the patient's age (see *Pediatric respiratory rates*).

This sign most commonly occurs in drug overdose or the advanced stages of neurologic and metabolic disorders that depress the brain's respiratory control centers (see *Understanding neurologic control of respiration*, page 38). It also can occur when pleuritic or thoracic cage pain causes voluntary restricted chest wall motion.

History questions

Explore the patient's problem by asking appropriate questions from this section.

• Did the bradypnea occur suddenly or gradually? If it occurred suddenly, did anything happen just before its onset?

• Is the patient experiencing any associated symptoms, such as seizures, headache, fatigue, weakness, nausea, vomiting, or diarrhea? Has he recently experienced flulike symptoms or upper respiratory infections?

• Does the patient have a chronic illness, such as diabetes, renal failure, chronic obstructive pulmonary disease, or thoracic cage disorder. Does he have a history of head trauma, brain tumor, neurologic infection, or cerebrovascular accident.

• Has the patient used nonprescription drugs, such as laxatives and antacids, or undergone treatments, such as GI suctioning and diuretic

Pediatric respiratory rates

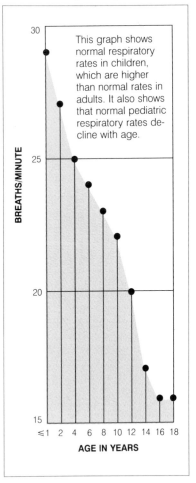

This graph shows normal respiratory rates in children, which are higher than normal rates in adults. It also shows that normal pediatric respiratory rates decline with age.

BREATHS/MINUTE

AGE IN YEARS

therapy, which might predispose him to acid-base imbalance.

• Investigate the possibility of drug overdose. Does the patient have a history of drug abuse? If so, try to determine which drugs the patient took, how much he took, and by which route.

• Is the patient taking any prescribed medications that can depress

Understanding neurologic control of respiration

The mechanical aspects of breathing are regulated by respiratory centers, groups of discrete neurons in the medulla and pons that function as a unit. In the medullary respiratory center, neurons associated with inspiration interact with neurons associated with expiration to control respiratory rate and depth. In the pons, two additional centers interact with the medullary center to regulate rhythm. The apneustic center stimulates inspiratory neurons in the medulla to precipitate inspiration; these, in turn, stimulate the pneumotaxic center to inhibit inspiration, allowing passive expiration.

Normally, the breathing mechanism is stimulated by increased carbon dioxide levels or decreased oxygen levels in the blood. Chemoreceptors in the medulla and in the carotid and aortic bodies respond to changes in partial pressure of carbon dioxide in arterial blood ($PaCO_2$), pH, and partial pressure of oxygen in arterial blood (PaO_2), signaling respiratory centers to adjust respiratory rate and depth.

Respiratory depression occurs when reduced cerebral perfusion inactivates respiratory center neurons, when changes in $PaCO_2$ and arterial blood pH affect chemoreceptor responsiveness, or when neuron responsiveness to $PaCO_2$ changes is reduced—for example, because of narcotic overdose.

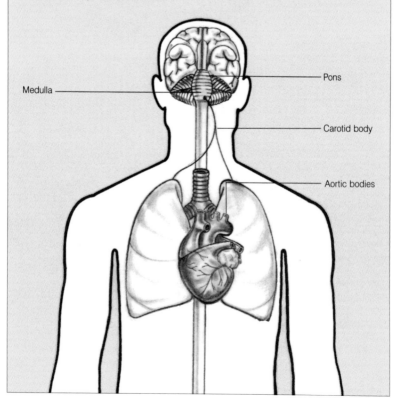

Medulla

Pons

Carotid body

Aortic bodies

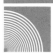 **Managing metabolic alkalosis and respiratory acidosis**

If you suspect that a patient with bradypnea has one of these two life-threatening disorders, you need to monitor his condition and take certain steps. Here's a rundown of what you should do.

Metabolic alkalosis
For this acid-base imbalance, monitor:
• level of consciousness
• neuromuscular function
• muscle strength and movement
• vital signs, especially respiratory rate and rhythm
• intake and output
• Chvostek's and Trousseau's signs
• appropriate laboratory values.
  Also, intervene as follows:
• Provide a safe physical environment.
• Institute seizure precautions.
• Provide enough stimuli to maintain orientation.
• Provide comfort measures for GI effects, such as vomiting and diarrhea.
• Administer prescribed fluids and medications.

Respiratory acidosis
For this condition, monitor:
• vital signs, especially respiratory rate and rhythm
• level of consciousness

• muscle strength, coordination, and movement
• patient comfort
• appropriate laboratory values
• skin for signs of hypoxia (a late sign).
  Also, intervene as follows:
• Maintain a safe, quiet environment with enough stimuli to maintain orientation.
• Encourage an amount of activity that's appropriate for the degree of hypoxia.
• Provide emotional support.
• Help the patient into a position that aids respiration.
• Use preventive pulmonary therapies to increase carbon dioxide removal by the lungs: turning, coughing, deep breathing, and suctioning.
• Administer oxygen when appropriate and as prescribed.
• Administer prescribed fluids and medications.

respirations, such as codeine, meperidine, phenobarbital, or other narcotic analgesics or sedatives? If so, is he taking them as ordered?

Physical examination
Base your assessment of the patient on the health history information you've collected.

Inspection. Observe the patient's respirations, noting rate and depth. Also, look for breathing difficulty and abnormal respiratory patterns, such as asymmetrical chest movement or paradoxical respirations.

Then assess his level of consciousness, noting belligerence, slow mental responses, restlessness, or disorientation. Does the patient have seizures, uncoordinated movements, or flapping tremors?

Check the arms and legs for needle marks, which may indicate drug abuse. Also inspect the skin for signs of dehydration, including dryness and poor turgor.

Palpation. Gently palpate the chest wall, sternum, and, if possible, the posterior thorax for crepitus and bone pieces associated with rib or

Respiratory acidosis: Recognizing predisposing conditions

This list shows conditions that can predispose a patient to respiratory acidosis as well as common causes of those conditions.

Airway obstruction

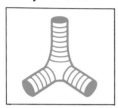

- Aspiration
- Foreign bodies
- Pulmonary embolus
- Severe bronchospasm
- Pulmonary edema
- Laryngeal edema

Muscle or nerve defects

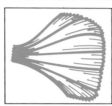

- Myasthenia gravis
- Guillain-Barré syndrome
- Poliomyelitis
- Botulism
- Spinal cord injury
- Hypokalemia
- Hyperkalemia

Pulmonary disease

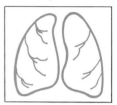

- Chronic obstructive pulmonary disease
- Smoke inhalation
- Pneumonia
- Atelectasis
- Asthma
- Interstitial lung disease
- Bronchitis
- Bronchiectasis

Respiratory center depression

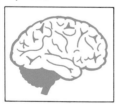

- Sedatives
- Chronic narcotic abuse
- Metabolic acidosis
- General anesthesia
- Increased intracranial pressure
- Medullary tumor
- Meningitis
- Vertebral artery embolus or thrombus

Thoracic cage disorders

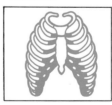

- Flail chest
- Pneumothorax
- Pickwickian syndrome
- Ankylosing spondylitis

sternum fractures. Evaluate motor function, comparing the right and left sides for strength and muscle tone. Palpate the muscles for evidence of neuromuscular irritability and tetany. Palpate the peripheral pulses for rate, rhythm, and intensity.

Percussion. Test deep tendon reflexes (brachial, ulnar, patellar, Achilles). Note any abnormal response.

Auscultation. Next, auscultate all lung fields for diminished or adventitious breath sounds, particularly crackles, rhonchi, and pleural friction rubs. Auscultate for heart sounds, noting any murmurs, pericardial friction rubs, or irregular rhythms. Check for hyperactive bowel sounds. Then monitor blood pressure and pulse pressure.

Life-threatening causes

Your assessment may lead you to suspect one or more of the following.

Metabolic alkalosis. A patient with this disorder may experience bradypnea along with increased neuromuscular irritability, tetany, seizures, altered level of consciousness, cardiac dysrhythmias, nausea, vomiting, and diarrhea. The patient may have a history of cystic fibrosis, hyperaldosteronism, Cushing's syndrome, hypokalemia, or hypercalcemia. Other predisposing factors include prolonged diarrhea, GI suctioning, diuretic therapy, laxative abuse, and excessive ingestion of licorice or alkalinizing salts, such as bicarbonate (see *Managing metabolic alkalosis and respiratory acidosis,* page 39).

Respiratory acidosis. In this disorder, bradypnea may be accompanied by an altered level of consciousness, ranging from slowed mental responses to coma, and apprehension, fatigue, weakness, and headache. The patient also may exhibit cardiac dysrhythmias, tachycardia, dyspnea, restlessness, flapping tremors, incoordination, or decreased reflexes. Cyanosis from hypoxia occurs late in this disorder. Predisposing factors include airway obstruction, respiratory center depression, respiratory neuromuscular defects, lung disease, and any thoracic cage disorder (see *Respiratory acidosis: Recognizing predisposing conditions*).

Other causes

Bradypnea also stems from certain disorders and drug overdoses that may not require prompt intervention.

Disorders. Respiratory center depression resulting from tumors or trauma to the medulla can cause bradypnea. Chest wall trauma and pleural disorders that cause pain on inspiration can cause voluntary guarding and bradypnea.

Drugs. Bradypnea also can result from respiratory center depression caused by an overdose of narcotic analgesics or, less commonly, sedatives, barbiturates, phenothiazines, or other central nervous system depressants.

Breath odor, fecal

Fecal breath odor represents a late diagnostic sign of an intestinal obstruction. If untreated, a complete obstruction of any part of the bowel can cause death within hours from vascular collapse and shock.

This danger sign accompanies fecal vomiting, which results when an obstructed or adynamic intestine attempts self-decompression by regurgitating its contents. Vigorous peristaltic waves propel bowel contents backward into the stomach. When the stomach fills with intestinal fluid, further reversed peristalsis results in vomiting. The odor of feculent vomitus lingers in the mouth.

History questions
Explore the patient's problem by asking appropriate questions from this section.
• Does the patient have abdominal pain? If so, have him describe its onset, duration, and location. Is the pain colicky, intense, persistent, or spasmodic?
• Has the patient experienced constipation, diarrhea, or leakage of stool? Find out when he had his last bowel movement, and have him describe its color and consistency.
• Is he nauseated? Ask if he's been vomiting; if so, how often? Have him describe the color, odor, amount, and consistency of the vomitus. Has the vomiting changed in any way since it started? Does he have any flulike symptoms, such as aches, malaise, or lethargy?
• Does the patient have a condition that could predispose him to bowel obstruction, including bowel cancer, volvulus, internal or external hernias, or diverticulitis. Ask about abdominal surgery or radiation therapy, which can cause adhesions.

Physical examination
Base your assessment of the patient on the health history information you've collected. Assess the abdomen, making sure you auscultate before percussing and palpating. Using this alternative sequence ensures that you don't affect the frequency or intensity of bowel sounds before you auscultate them.

Inspection. Assess abdominal contour and note any surgical scars. Also look for distention, visible peristaltic waves, or distended bowel loops. Take a baseline measurement of abdominal girth and remeasure regularly; an increase may indicate bleeding. Observe the patient's respirations, noting rate and depth. Also, look for breathing difficulty and abnormal respiratory patterns.

Auscultation. Using the diaphragm of your stethoscope, auscultate the patient's bowel sounds. Then monitor blood pressure and pulse pressure.

Palpation. As you palpate the abdomen, note any tenderness, rigidity, or abdominal masses. Palpate peripheral pulses, noting their rate, rhythm, and intensity.

Percussion. Next, gently percuss the abdomen. You'll hear tympanic sounds over gas pockets and dull sounds over fluid-filled areas.

Life-threatening causes
Your assessment may lead you to suspect one or more of the following.

Distal small-bowel obstruction. In late-stage obstruction, fecal breath odor occurs along with abdominal distention, tympanic percussion notes, borborygmus, and persistent paroxysmal, colicky epigastric or periumbilical pain. Typically, the patient will have hyperactive, high-pitched bowel sounds with almost a musical quality. These change to hypoactive or absent sounds as the obstruction progresses. Aches, malaise, drowsiness, polydipsia, and diarrhea or constipation also may occur. Fever, hypotension, tachycardia, and rebound tenderness may indicate bowel perforation. The patient may have a history of abdominal surgery, radiation therapy, or internal or external hernias.

Large-bowel obstruction. In this disorder, fecal vomiting with fecal breath odor occurs as a rare late sign. Typically, symptoms develop more slowly than in small-bowel obstruction. Colicky abdominal pain begins suddenly, followed by continuous hypogastric pain. Marked abdominal distention and tenderness and tympanic percussion sounds occur. You may be able to see loops of the large bowel through the abdominal wall. Bowel sounds will be less frequent and lower-pitched than in small-bowel obstruction. Although constipation always develops, bowel movements may continue up to 3 days after a complete obstruction occurs because of the stool remaining below the obstruction. Leakage of stool is common with partial obstruction. The patient may have a history of volvulus or diverticulitis.

Other cause
Fecal breath odor also results from gastrojejunocolic fistula, which doesn't require immediate intervention.

Breath odor, fruity

Fruity breath odor results from respiratory elimination of excess acetone. This sign characteristically occurs in ketoacidosis — a potentially life-threatening condition caused by an excessive catabolism of fats for cellular energy when usable carbohydrates aren't available.

Ketoacidosis occurs when insulin levels aren't sufficient to transport glucose into the cells, as in diabetes mellitus, or when glucose is unavailable and hepatic glycogen stores are depleted, as in low-carbohydrate diets and malnutrition. Lacking glucose, the cells burn fat faster than enzymes can handle the acidic end products, ketones. As a result, the ketones (acetone, beta-hydroxybutyric acid, and acetoacetic acid) accumulate in the blood and urine.

To compensate for the increased acidity, Kussmaul's respirations expel carbon dioxide with enough acetone to flavor the breath. Eventually, this compensatory mechanism fails, producing ketoacidosis.

History questions
Explore the patient's problem by asking appropriate questions from this section.
• When did the patient or a member of his family first notice the fruity breath odor. Find out if and when they noticed a change in his breathing pattern — for example, to deep, rapid respirations. Ask about other associated symptoms, such as increased thirst, frequent urination, weakness, fatigue, and abdominal pain.
• Has the patient recently lost weight? If so, how much and over what period? Ask the patient about his usual diet and find out whether he's been restricting his carbohydrate intake.
• Does the patient have cancer, severe infection, or malabsorption syndrome? Does he have a history of anorexia nervosa or bulimia? Does he have a history of diabetes mellitus? If so, ask about stress,

past and current infections, and noncompliance with therapy—the most common causes of ketoacidosis in diabetics.

Physical examination

Base your assessment of the patient on the health history information you've collected. Be sure to auscultate the abdomen before percussing and palpating. Using this alternative sequence ensures that you don't affect the frequency and intensity of bowel sounds before you auscultate them.

Inspection. Observe the entire body for obvious muscle wasting and dry, scaly skin. Check the abdomen for distention. Then observe the patient's respirations, noting rate and depth. Does he have difficulty breathing? What about abnormal respiratory patterns, particularly Kussmaul's respirations?

Auscultation. First, auscultate the heart for a rapid or slow rate. Then auscultate the abdomen for hyperactive bowel sounds and abdominal masses. To detect orthostatic hypotension, check the patient's blood pressure with him supine and sitting. Also, be sure to monitor his blood pressure and pulse pressure.

Palpation. Now, palpate the patient's muscles for wasting or flaccidity. Then palpate the abdomen for pain or tenderness. Assess for poor skin turgor and dry mucous membranes—indications of dehydration. Also, check his peripheral pulses, noting their rate, rhythm, and intensity.

Percussion. Check for flaccid reflexes and percuss the abdomen to detect pain or tenderness.

Life-threatening causes

Your assessment may lead you to suspect one or more of the following.

Diabetic ketoacidosis. Fruity breath odor often occurs as the ketoacidosis develops over 1 or 2 days. Associated signs and symptoms include polydipsia, polyuria, polyphagia, weak and rapid pulse, weight loss, weakness, fatigue, nausea, vomiting, and abdominal pain and distention. As the disorder progresses, Kussmaul's respirations, orthostatic hypotension, flaccid reflexes, dehydration, tachycardia, confusion, and stupor occur. Symptoms progressively worsen and may lead to coma. The patient may have a history of diabetes mellitus.

Starvation ketoacidosis. In this disorder, fruity breath odor typically is accompanied by Kussmaul's respirations, anorexia, and weight loss. The patient also may have orthostatic hypotension, bradycardia, abdominal distention, dry scaly skin, poor wound healing, muscle and tissue wasting, and possible disorientation progressing to stupor and coma. He may complain of weakness, fatigue, abdominal pain, a sore tongue, and nausea. His history may reveal rapid weight loss, anorexia nervosa, or bulimia.

Carpopedal spasm

Violent, painful contraction of the hand and foot muscles, carpopedal spasm is an important sign of tetany. This condition, characterized by increased neuromuscular excitation and sustained muscle contraction, is commonly associated with hypocalcemia.

Carpopedal spasm requires prompt evaluation and intervention of the underlying cause. If untreated, it can lead to laryngospasm, seizures, cardiac dysrhythmias, and cardiac and respiratory arrest.

History questions

Explore the patient's problem by asking appropriate questions from this section.
• Ask when the spasms started and how long they last. How much pain do they cause? Has the patient experienced similar spasms before?
• Does the patient have any other signs and symptoms of hypocalcemia? Ask about numbness and tingling of the fingertips, feet, or mouth; other muscle cramps or spasms; nausea; vomiting; abdominal pain; fatigue; and palpitations.
• Has the patient or a family member noticed changes in his behavior or personality?
• Has the patient undergone neck or GI surgery? What about multiple blood transfusions or phosphate infusion? Does he have a history of hypoparathyroidism, pseudohypoparathyroidism, calcium or vitamin D deficiency, malabsorption syndrome, acute pancreatitis, bone malignancy, or renal disease?
• Is he taking any medications that could lead to calcium or magnesium deficiency, such as a loop diuretic, antibiotics, dactinomycin, or plicamycin?

Physical examination

Base your assessment of the patient on the health history information you've collected. Maintain a quiet, calm environment to reduce the patient's anxiety as you proceed with the examination.

Inspection. Observe for muscle seizures, twitching, or evidence of extreme anxiety. Inspect the patient for signs of chronic calcium deficiency — dry skin, brittle nails, and alopecia. Observe the patient's respirations, noting rate and depth. Does he have difficulty breathing? Abnormal respiratory patterns?

Palpation. Next, palpate the muscle groups for weakness and atrophy or sustained muscular contractions. Also, palpate the peripheral pulses for rate, rhythm, and intensity.

Percussion. To detect muscle cramps associated with hypocalcemia, percuss the muscle groups. Percuss over the facial nerve to test for Chvostek's sign (see *Recognizing carpopedal spasm,* page 46).

Auscultation. Assess for a partial airway obstruction by auscultating all lung fields for adventitious breath sounds, particularly crowing noises and wheezing. Then monitor the patient's blood pressure and pulse pressure.

Life-threatening causes

Your assessment may lead you to suspect this disorder.

Hypocalcemic tetany. Serum calcium deficiency and the resulting neuromuscular irritability produce carpopedal spasm. Other signs and symptoms include muscle weakness, twitching, and cramping; laryngospasm and stridor; and, mainly in children, tonic-clonic seizures. You also may note paresthesia of the fingers, toes, and circumoral area; hyperreflexia; chorea; fatigue; palpitations; and positive Chvostek's and Trousseau's signs, as well as signs of the underlying disorder.

Typically, the patient has an underlying problem predisposing him to hypocalcemia, such as

Recognizing carpopedal spasm

What exactly does carpopedal spasm look like? You'll see adduction of the thumb over the palm, followed by flexion of the metacarpophalangeal joints, extension of the interphalangeal joints (fingers together), adduction of the hyperextended fingers, and flexion of the wrist and elbow joints. Similar effects occur in the joints of the feet.

On assessment, you'll also be able to elicit two abnormal muscle spasms associated with hypocalcemia—Chvostek's sign and Trousseau's sign.

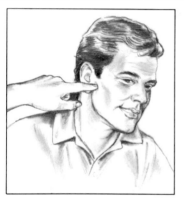

To elicit *Chvostek's sign*, tap one finger in front of your patient's ear at the angle of the jaw, over the facial nerve. Muscle contracture is considered a positive Chvostek's sign.

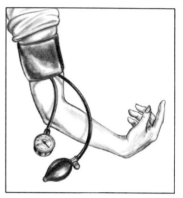

To elicit *Trousseau's sign*, apply a blood pressure cuff to the patient's arm just above the antecubital area, then inflate the cuff until you've occluded the arm's blood supply. A carpal spasm is considered a positive Trousseau's sign.

malabsorption from recent GI surgery, hypoparathyroidism, vitamin D deficiency, acute pancreatitis, or metastatic bone malignancy. Hypocalcemic tetany also stems from increased serum phosphate concentration resulting from leukemia, chemotherapy, or phosphate infusion.

Other causes

Certain causes of carpopedal spasm aren't life-threatening and may not require emergency intervention.

Disorders. Hyperventilation and respiratory alkalosis can produce tetany with carpopedal spasm in a patient who has a normal serum calcium level. Having the patient breathe into a paper bag will alleviate spasm and any other symptoms.

Drugs. Loop diuretics, antibiotics, dactinomycin, or plicamycin can cause a calcium or magnesium deficiency, predisposing a patient to hypocalcemic tetany.

Multiple blood transfusions can cause hypocalcemic tetany because the citrate in stored blood binds with serum calcium.

Surgery. Parathyroidectomy can cause hypocalcemia with carpopedal spasm, as may surgical procedures that impair calcium absorption, such as ileostomy and gastric resection with gastrojejunostomy.

Chest pain

Chest pain most commonly results from ischemic or inflammatory disorders affecting thoracic or abdominal structures—the heart, pleurae, lungs, gallbladder, pancreas, or stomach. But it can also result from musculoskeletal and hematologic disorders, anxiety, and drug therapy. What's more, chest pain may be caused or aggravated by stress, anxiety, exertion, deep breathing, or eating certain foods. (For more information, see *Understanding cardiac and pleural chest pain,* pages 48 and 49.)

Chest pain can arise suddenly or gradually and can radiate to the arms, neck, jaw, or back. It may be steady or intermittent, mild or acute. And it can range in character from a sharp shooting sensation to a feeling of heaviness, fullness, or even indigestion.

History questions
Explore the patient's problem by asking appropriate questions from this section.
• Ask about chest pain's onset. Did the pain start suddenly or gradually? Is it more severe or frequent now than when it started? Sudden, severe chest pain requires prompt evaluation and treatment—it may indicate a life-threatening disorder.
• Is the pain localized or diffused? Does it radiate to the neck, jaw, arms, or back? Have the patient describe it: Is it a dull, aching, pressurelike sensation? A sharp, stabbing, knifelike pain? Does he feel it on the surface or deep inside?
• Is the pain constant or intermittent? If it's intermittent, how long does each episode last? Does movement, exertion, breathing, changing positions, or eating certain foods worsen or relieve the pain?
• Find out if he's felt similar pain before. If so, does he take medication, such as nitroglycerin, to relieve it?
• Ask about any associated symptoms. Has the patient experienced any syncope, palpitations, weakness, or transient paralysis (especially of the legs)? What about headache, light-headedness, myalgia, or fatigue? Has he or his family noticed any changes in his level of consciousness? Does he feel any abdominal pain? What about nausea, vomiting, anorexia, or epistaxis?
• Does the patient have dyspnea, particularly on exertion? A cough—either productive or nonproductive? If the cough is productive, describe the sputum color and consistency.
• Does he have a recent history of myocardial infarction (MI), congestive heart failure (CHF), cardiogenic shock, or congestive cardiomyopathy? Also ask about recent upper respiratory infection, thrombophlebitis, hip or leg fractures, prolonged bed rest, or pregnancy.
• Does the patient have a history of pulmonary disease; blunt or penetrating chest trauma; intestinal, renal, or connective tissue disease; lung cancer; or sickle cell anemia?

Understanding cardiac and pleural chest pain

Although chest pain is one of the most common symptoms of heart disease, it doesn't always originate in the heart. It can, for instance, result from a pulmonary, GI, or musculoskeletal problem.

In the following illustrations, you'll see how two common types of chest pain develop.

Cardiac chest pain
Atherosclerosis, arterial vasospasm or thrombus, or suddenly increased myocardial oxygen demands (for example, during stress) may cause inadequate coronary perfusion. The reduced blood flow diminishes oxygen delivery to the heart, causing tissue ischemia and forcing the heart to shift to anaerobic metabolism, which produces lactic acid as a by-product. The accumulation of lactic acid, or any stimuli that causes tissue ischemia, may activate pain receptors in the affected area.

Pleural chest pain
Viral infection of the pleura may also cause chest pain. Such infection leads to inflammation, with subsequent swelling and congestion that hamper pleural fluid flow. As a result, friction increases between the pleural surfaces, causing irritation and activating pain receptors in the parietal pleura.

Pain transmission
Pleural and cardiac pain receptors relay the pain impulse through the dorsal sensory route and the spinal cord to the thalamus, where pain is perceived. The cerebral cortex further differentiates the degree, type, and location of pain.

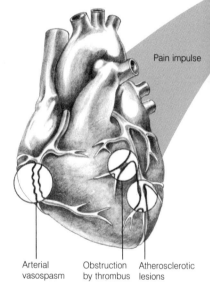

CORONARY ARTERIES

Pain impulse

Arterial vasospasm

Obstruction by thrombus

Atherosclerotic lesions

• Has the patient ever undergone cardiac or other surgery? Has he recently had subclavian vein cannulation or received mechanical ventilation under pressure?

• Is the patient taking any medication or has he recently changed dosage or schedule? Oral contraceptives can predispose a patient to thrombophlebitis and pulmonary embolism; procainamide or hydralazine can cause pericarditis; nonsteroidal anti-inflammatory drugs, aspirin, or corticosteroids can lead to GI ulceration; and octreotide can cause gallstones.

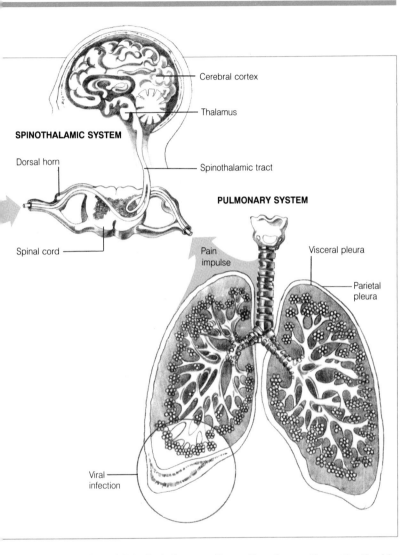

SPINOTHALAMIC SYSTEM

Cerebral cortex

Thalamus

Dorsal horn

Spinothalamic tract

PULMONARY SYSTEM

Spinal cord

Pain impulse

Visceral pleura

Parietal pleura

Viral infection

• Does the patient drink alcohol or use illicit drugs—especially cocaine, which can precipitate an MI.

Physical examination
Base your assessment of the patient on the health history information you've collected.

Inspection. Assess the patient's skin temperature and color, noting cyanosis, pallor, mottling below the waist, peripheral edema, diaphoresis, and prolonged capillary refill time (greater than 2 seconds). Look too for jugular vein distention, tracheal deviation, or facial edema.

Then observe the patient's respirations, noting the rate and depth. Does he have difficulty breathing? Do you see abnormal respiratory patterns?

Assess the patient's neurologic status, noting any anxiety, restlessness, dizziness, or altered level of consciousness. If the patient has produced sputum, check its color and consistency.

Palpation. As you palpate the lungs, neck, and abdomen, note any vocal or tactile fremitus, asymmetrical chest expansion, subcutaneous crepitation, tracheal deviation, masses, or tender areas. Palpate peripheral pulses, noting the rate, rhythm, and intensity. Also check for weak or absent femoral or pedal pulses and decreased carotid artery pulse.

Percussion. Now, percuss over the affected lung to detect dullness.

Auscultation. First, auscultate the lungs for pleural friction rubs, crackles, rhonchi, wheezes, diminished or absent breath sounds, whispered pectoriloquy, hyperresonance, or tympany. Next, auscultate the heart for murmurs, clicks, gallops, or pericardial friction rub. With the bell of the stethoscope, auscultate over the abdominal aorta for abdominal bruits.

Monitor the patient's blood pressure and pulse pressure. Be sure to measure blood pressure in the arms and legs, noting any deviations.

Life-threatening causes
Your assessment may lead you to suspect one or more of the following.

Aortic aneurysm (dissecting). Chest pain usually begins suddenly and is severe at onset. The patient describes an excruciating tearing, ripping, or stabbing pain in the chest and neck radiating to the upper back, abdomen, and lower back. (Dull or absent pain may reflect compromised neurologic function.) The patient also may have abdominal tenderness and a palpable abdominal mass, tachycardia, heart murmurs, pericardial friction rub, systolic bruits, jugular vein distention, and tracheal deviation.

Other signs and symptoms include syncope, altered level of consciousness, weakness or transient paralysis of an extremity (particularly the legs), systemic hypotension with ascending aortic dissection or hypertension with thoracic aortic dissection, lower blood pressure in the legs than in the arms, prolonged capillary refill time, weak or absent femoral or pedal pulses, and decreased pulses in one or both carotid arteries. The skin may be pale, cool, diaphoretic, and mottled below the waist. The patient may have a history of cardiovascular disease or chest pain.

Mediastinitis. In this disorder, inflammation or infection produces severe retrosternal chest pain that radiates to the epigastrium, back, or shoulder and may worsen with breathing, coughing, or sneezing. Typically, the pain is accompanied by chills, fever, and dysphagia. Puffiness of the neck and face, cyanosis, headache, epistaxis, and light-headedness indicate superior vena cava involvement. The patient's recent history may include endotracheal intubation or episodes of severe vomiting or aspiration. Or he may have swallowed a foreign body. His history may also include esophagoscopy or a chronic disease (such as histoplasmosis, silicosis, or systemic lupus erythematosus), or drug therapy with methysergide, amiodarone, or bleomycin.

Myocardial infarction. The patient will feel severe, crushing substernal chest pain that may radiate to his left arm, jaw, neck, abdomen, or shoulder blades. The pain won't be relieved by rest or nitroglycerin and may be accompanied by pallor, clammy skin, dyspnea, diaphoresis, nausea, vomiting, anxiety, restlessness, weakness, dizziness, and a feeling of impending doom. The patient may develop hypotension or hypertension, an atrial gallop, murmurs, pericardial friction rub, and crackles. He may have a history of heart disease, hypertension, hypercholesterolemia, or cocaine abuse. (For more information, see *Managing an MI,* page 52.)

Myocardial ischemia. Oxygen-deficient myocardial cells produce a feeling of tightness or pressure in the chest that the patient may describe as pain or a sensation of indigestion or expansion. Usually, the pain occurs in the retrosternal region over a palm-sized or larger area. It may radiate to the neck, jaw, and arms—classically, to the inner aspect of the left arm. Anginal pain tends to begin gradually, build to a peak, then slowly subside. Lasting from 2 to 10 minutes, the pain may occur at rest or be provoked by exertion, emotional stress, or a heavy meal. Accompanying signs and symptoms may include dyspnea, nausea, vomiting, tachycardia, dizziness, diaphoresis, belching, or palpitations. You may hear an atrial gallop (S_4) or murmur during an anginal episode. The patient's history may include cardiovascular disease and previous episodes of chest pain relieved by nitroglycerin.

Pericarditis. Pericardial inflammation produces sudden, persistent precordial or retrosternal chest pain aggravated by deep breathing, coughing, position changes, and, occasionally, by swallowing. Commonly, the pain is sharp or cutting and radiates to the shoulder and neck. Accompanying signs and symptoms may include pericardial friction rub, fever, tachycardia, and dyspnea. The patient may have a history of bacterial, viral, or fungal disease; recent MI; recent cardiac surgery; blunt or penetrating chest trauma; uremia; connective tissue disease; serum sickness; or use of drugs associated with pericarditis, such as procainamide or hydralazine.

Pneumonia. Inflamed pleurae produce pleuritic chest pain increasing on deep inspiration and accompanied by shaking chills and fever. The patient will have a dry or productive cough, depending on the stage and type of pneumonia; sputum may be discolored and foul-smelling. Other signs and symptoms may include decreased breath sounds, crackles, rhonchi, dull percussion sounds, whispered pectoriloquy, tachycardia, tachypnea, myalgia, fatigue, headache, dyspnea, abdominal pain, anorexia, cyanosis, and diaphoresis. The patient may have a history of smoking, chronic obstructive pulmonary disease, or exposure to hazardous fumes, air pollution, or a contagious organism.

Pneumothorax. Lung collapse produces sudden, sharp, severe chest pain that's often unilateral and increases with chest movement. Pain located centrally and radiating

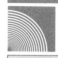

Managing an MI

If, after your assessment, you suspect that the patient is having a myocardial infarction (MI), notify the doctor immediately. Then take these steps.

Initial interventions
Administer oxygen at 2 to 4 liters/minute. Then insert an I.V. line for emergency drugs. Prepare to obtain venous blood samples for laboratory tests such as cardiac enzyme studies, electrolyte levels, clotting profile, and a complete blood count.

Obtain a 12-lead electrocardiogram and place the patient on a cardiac monitor to detect life-threatening dysrhythmias. Keep the crash cart nearby.

Place the patient in a position that enhances ventilations.

Administering medications
To dilate the coronary arteries and improve blood flow, you may give sublingual nitroglycerin or isosorbide dinitrate, as ordered. Morphine, meperidine, or hydromorphone can be given I.V. to ease the patient's pain. If these drugs don't work, nitroglycerin may be administered by continuous drip. To reduce coronary spasm and help ease pain, verapamil or nifedipine may be given. Depending on when the pain began, a thrombolytic—streptokinase, alteplase, or anistreplase—may be given to dissolve the clot causing the obstruction. These thrombolytics are most effective when given within 6 hours of the onset of symptoms.

Checking for complications
Monitor the patient for complications of the MI. Take his vital signs every 15 to 30 minutes until he's stable. Keep assessing his level of consciousness—a sensitive indicator of tissue perfusion and oxygenation.

If cardiogenic shock develops, you'll note changes in the patient's level of consciousness, tachycardia, systolic blood pressure that's less than 80 mm Hg or 30 mm Hg less than baseline, narrowed pulse pressure, diminished Korotkoff's sounds, and pale, cool, clammy skin. In a patient with these signs and symptoms, a central line may be inserted to monitor cardiac output. An intra-aortic balloon pump may be used to reduce left ventricular work load and improve coronary perfusion.

Correcting dysrhythmias
Dysrhythmias frequently occur after an MI because of myocardial ischemia and irritability. Expect to administer lidocaine for premature ventricular contractions, atropine for symptomatic bradycardia, and isoproterenol for complete heart block. For a heart block, the doctor may also insert a temporary pacemaker. Supraventricular tachycardias (atrial fibrillation, atrial flutter, or paroxysmal atrial tachycardia with rapid ventricular response) may respond to carotid massage or Valsalva's maneuver. If not, verapamil, propranolol, or digoxin may be given I.V. If these drugs fail to correct the dysrhythmia, cardioversion may be ordered.

Providing emotional support
Remember, the MI patient will probably be afraid that he's going to die. The I.V. lines and monitors will only worsen his anxiety. By providing emotional support and explaining procedures thoroughly to him, you can decrease his anxiety and stress, thereby reducing his myocardial oxygen consumption.

to the neck may mimic an MI. After the pain begins, dyspnea and cyanosis worsen progressively. Breath sounds are decreased or absent on the affected side, accompanied by hyperresonant or tympanic percussion sounds, subcutaneous crepitation, and decreased vocal fremitus. Asymmetrical chest expansion, accessory muscle use, nonproductive cough, tachypnea, tachycardia, anxiety, and restlessness also commonly occur. The patient's history may include recent subclavian vein cannulation, chronic obstructive pulmonary disease, lung malignancy, mechanical ventilation under pressure, or diagnostic or therapeutic procedures involving the thorax.

Pulmonary embolism. Typically, the patient experiences sudden dyspnea with an intense angina-like or pleuritic ischemic pain aggravated by deep breathing and thoracic movement. Other findings may include anxiety, tachycardia, tachypnea, cough (which may produce blood-tinged sputum), low-grade fever, restlessness, diaphoresis, crackles, pleural friction rub, diffuse wheezing, and dull percussion sounds. The patient also may experience signs of circulatory collapse (weak, rapid pulse; hypotension), signs of cerebral ischemia (transient unconsciousness, coma, seizures), signs of hypoxia (restlessness), and — particularly in elderly patients — hemiplegia and other focal neurologic deficits.

Less common signs include massive hemoptysis, chest splinting, and leg edema. A patient with a large embolus may have cyanosis and distended neck veins. The patient's history may reveal thrombophlebitis of the deep systemic veins, hip or leg fractures, acute MI,

CHF, cardiogenic shock, congestive cardiomyopathy, pregnancy, or use of oral contraceptives.

Other causes
Certain causes of chest pain may not signal the need for immediate intervention.

Disorders. Many disorders can produce chest pain, including severe anxiety, blastomycosis, bronchitis, cardiomyopathy, Chinese restaurant syndrome (a benign reaction to monosodium glutamate), cholecystitis, coccidioidomycosis, costochondral osteochondritis, distention of the splenic flexure, esophageal spasm, herpes zoster (shingles), and hiatal hernia. Chest pain can also stem from interstitial lung disease, Legionnaires' disease, lung abscess, lung cancer, mitral valve prolapse, muscle strain, nocardiosis, peptic ulcer, pleurisy, pleuritis, pneumomediastinum, psittacosis, pulmonary actinomycosis, pulmonary hypertension (primary), rib fracture, sickle cell disease, thoracic outlet syndrome, and tuberculosis.

Drugs. Abrupt withdrawal of beta blockers can cause rebound angina in a patient with coronary heart disease — especially if he's received prolonged high-dose therapy.

Cheyne-Stokes respirations

This breathing pattern consists of a waxing and waning period of hyperpnea alternating with a shorter period of apnea (see *Understanding Cheyne-Stokes respirations,* page 54). Cheyne-Stokes respirations can

Understanding Cheyne-Stokes respirations

These illustrations show you the difference between normal respirations and Cheyne-Stokes respirations.

Eupnea
With normal respirations, the rate and rhythm are regular. For adults and teenagers, the normal rate is 12 to 20 breaths/minute; for children ages 2 to 12, 20 to 30 breaths/minute; and for newborns, 30 to 50 breaths/minute.

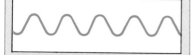

Cheyne-Stokes respirations
With Cheyne-Stokes respirations, breathing gradually becomes faster and deeper than normal, then slower, over a 30- to 170-second period. These periods alternate with 20- to 60-second periods of apnea, indicated by the flat baseline.

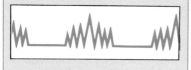

occur normally in people who live at high altitudes and in elderly people during sleep. Most often, however, this breathing pattern indicates a dysfunction of the respiratory centers in the brain stem, in which the response to carbon dioxide levels fluctuates. Cheyne-Stokes is the most common pattern of periodic breathing.

History questions
Explore the patient's problem by asking appropriate questions from this section.

• How long has the patient been breathing like this? Has he ever experienced this breathing pattern before, particularly at night? Does he ever wake up during the night with a feeling of breathlessness?
• Investigate any associated symptoms. Has the patient experienced any fatigue or weakness? Any vision changes, such as blurring, diplopia, or photophobia? What about productive or nonproductive cough? If the cough is productive, have him describe sputum color and consistency.
• Ask about recent head trauma or systemic infection and any history of diabetes mellitus, liver disease, renal failure, brain tumor, seizures, hypertension, or cardiac disease. Also find out if he's taking any medications — especially narcotics, hypnotics, or barbiturates. Large doses of these drugs can bring on Cheyne-Stokes respirations.

Physical examination
Base your assessment of the patient on the health history information you've collected.

Inspection. Observe the patient's respirations, noting the rate and depth. Does he have difficulty breathing? What about abnormal respiratory patterns? Time the hyperpneic and apneic episodes for 3 or 4 minutes to obtain a baseline.

Inspect the patient's skin and mucous membranes for edema, diaphoresis, or cyanosis. If he's experienced head or neck trauma, check for raccoon eyes, Battle's sign, and otorrhea. Observe his motor function and evaluate his muscle strength and tone. Be sure to compare one side with the other.

Palpation. If you suspect a skull fracture, gently palpate the patient's head for crepitus or depression. Then palpate his peripheral pulses, noting the rate, rhythm, and intensity.

Percussion. Check the patient's deep tendon reflexes, comparing the right and left sides. Percuss his abdomen, particularly for hepatomegaly.

Auscultation. Next, auscultate all lung fields for adventitious breath sounds, such as crackles and rhonchi. As you auscultate the patient's heart sounds, note any murmurs or abnormal sounds, particularly ventricular gallops. Then check his blood pressure for alternating loud and soft Korotkoff's sounds. Also, monitor his blood pressure and pulse pressure.

Life-threatening disorders

Your assessment may lead you to suspect one or more of the following.

Increased intracranial pressure. Cheyne-Stokes respirations signal deteriorating brain function and, in patients at risk, imminent transtentorial herniation. This danger sign occurs with bradycardia and widened pulse pressure and typically is preceded by elevated systolic blood pressure, tachycardia, tachypnea or apneustic respirations, progressive loss of consciousness, hypertension, seizures, headache, vomiting, impaired or unequal motor movement, and visual disturbances (blurring, diplopia, photophobia, and pupillary changes). The patient's history may reveal recent head trauma or systemic infection, brain tumor, or underlying metabolic or cardiac disease.

Left ventricular failure. Cheyne-Stokes respirations may occur at night, waking the patient and causing him to complain of dyspnea. Related findings may include fatigue, weakness, normal or low blood pressure, pulsus alternans, ventricular gallop, alternating loud and soft Korotkoff's sounds, tachycardia, tachypnea, and bilateral crackles. You may also note neck vein distention, prolonged capillary refill time, dependent edema, hepatomegaly, pallor or cyanosis, diaphoresis, and anxiety. The patient may have a cough. Usually, it'll be nonproductive, but sometimes a patient's cough will produce clear or blood-tinged sputum. Typically, the health history reveals preexisting cardiac disease accompanied by atherosclerosis, which further reduces cerebral blood flow.

Other causes

Certain causes of Cheyne-Stokes respirations may not require immediate intervention.

Disorders. A patient with chronic obstructive pulmonary disease may experience Cheyne-Stokes respirations during non-rapid-eye-movement sleep.

Drugs. Large doses of hypnotics, narcotics, or barbiturates can cause Cheyne-Stokes respirations.

Conjunctival injection

A common ocular sign associated with inflammation, conjunctival injection is an irregular redness of the conjunctiva due to hyperemia. This redness can be diffuse, localized, or peripheral — or it may encircle a clear cornea. In most cases, conjunctival injection results

Managing burns to the eye

When a patient suffers a burn to the eye, your main priorities are to determine what substance caused the burn and if he's wearing contact lenses. If he is, remove them. Then, as ordered, instill anesthetic eyedrops, as shown.

INSTILLING EYEDROPS

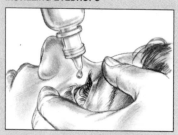

To flush out a caustic substance, continuously irrigate with normal saline solution as shown below. If the patient has an acidic chemical burn, keep flushing until eye pH returns to normal—a pH of 7. You should irrigate for 10 minutes before checking the pH with litmus paper. If the patient has alkaline chemical burns, use citric or boric acid instead of normal saline solution.

IRRIGATING THE EYE

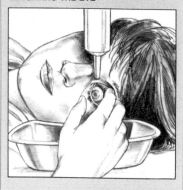

from bacterial or viral conjunctivitis. But it also can signal a severe ocular disorder that, if untreated, may lead to permanent blindness.

History questions

Explore the patient's problem by asking appropriate questions from this section.

• Ask when the patient first noticed the redness in his eye. Was the onset associated with exposure to intense heat, such as a flash fire, a hot object, ultraviolet rays from a sunlamp, or infrared rays or welding? What about exposure to aerosols (such as commercial solvents, ammonia, paints, or tear gas), caustic substances (such as battery acid, bleach, or other chemicals), allergens, or toxins?

• Does the patient feel any associated pain? If so, when did it begin and where is it? Is it constant or intermittent? Mild or severe?

• Ask about other accompanying symptoms, such as photophobia, excessive tearing, and decreased visual acuity. Does the patient feel any itching or burning? Does he feel as though a foreign body is in the eye?

• Does the patient have a history of eye disease? Has he recently been exposed to contagious bacterial, fungal, viral, or protozoal organisms?

Physical examination

Base your assessment of the patient on the health history information you've collected.

Inspection. Determine the location and the severity of the conjunctival injection. Is it circumcorneal or localized? Peripheral or diffuse?

Note any deviations in corneal color, conjunctival or lid edema, ocular deviation, conjunctival follicles, ptosis, or exophthalmos. Also note the type and amount of any discharge.

Check whether the size of pupils is equal and how they react to light. Note any vision changes, such as blurred vision or decreased acuity.

Vision-threatening causes

Your assessment may lead you to suspect one or more of the following.

Burns. In this ocular emergency, diffuse conjunctival injection occurs, but severe pain is the prominent symptom. The patient also may experience increased tearing, photophobia, blepharospasm, and decreased visual acuity in the affected eye. The cornea may appear gray, and the affected pupil may be smaller than the unaffected one. The history will reveal recent exposure to intense heat, smoke, aerosols, or chemicals. (For more information, see *Managing burns to the eye.*)

Corneal ulcer. Bacterial, viral, and fungal corneal ulcers may produce diffuse conjunctival injection that increases in the circumcorneal area. Associated findings typically include severe photophobia, severe pain in and around the eye that's aggravated by blinking, increased tearing, markedly decreased visual acuity, and copious and purulent ocular discharge and crusting. If the patient has associated iritis, you'll also note corneal opacities and an abnormal pupillary response to light. The patient's history may include recent eye trauma, possibly from contact lenses, or recent exposure to contagious organisms, allergens, or toxins.

Other causes

Conjunctival injection also results from conditions that may not require immediate intervention. Most often, this ocular sign is caused by minor eye irritation from lack of sleep, overuse of contact lenses, exposure to environmental irritants, or rubbing the eyes. It also may result from an astigmatism; a corneal abrasion or erosion; dacryoadenitis; episcleritis; intraocular foreign bodies; iritis; keratoconjunctivitis; ocular lacerations; ocular tumors; ophthalmitis; Stevens-Johnson syndrome; uveitis; or allergic, bacterial, fungal, or viral conjunctivitis.

At birth, an infant can develop self-limiting chemical conjunctivitis from ocular instillation of silver nitrate. Two to 5 days after birth, an infant may develop bacterial conjunctivitis from contamination in the birth canal. An infant with congenital syphilis will have prominent conjunctival injection and grayish pink corneas.

Constipation

Constipation is defined as small, infrequent, and difficult bowel movements. Normal bowel movements vary from twice a day to once every 3 days. So a diagnosis of constipation depends, in part, on the patient's normal elimination pattern.

Most commonly, constipation occurs when the urge to defecate is suppressed and the muscles associated with bowel movements remain contracted. In some cases, however, it signals life-threatening bowel obstruction or ischemia.

History questions

Explore the patient's problem by asking appropriate questions from this section.

• Have the patient describe the frequency, amount, and consistency of his bowel movements. How long has he been constipated? Is he able to pass any flatus?

• Does he feel any pain related to constipation? If so, when did it start? Is it localized or generalized, constant or intermittent? Does it radiate to any areas? Do attempts at passing stool or flatus worsen or help relieve the pain?

• Is the patient experiencing palpitations or a fever? What about anorexia, nausea, or vomiting? If the patient has been vomiting, is the vomitus feculent or bilious?

• Have the patient describe a typical day's menu and activities. Ask about any recent changes in eating habits, medication or alcohol use, and physical activity. Has he been under any emotional stress lately? Has constipation affected his home or social life? Also ask about his job. A sedentary or stressful job can contribute to constipation.

• Explore the patient's history for GI, neurologic, or metabolic disorders; internal or external hernias; abdominal surgery; or radiation therapy. Has he recently experienced an episode of hypoperfusion, such as congestive heart failure (CHF), cardiac dysrhythmias, or hypotension?

• Has he recently undergone any diagnostic tests in which he had to swallow barium? Obtain a medication history, noting whether he's using codeine, meperidine, and other narcotic analgesics or sedatives. Also investigate his use of over-the-counter preparations, such as antacids, laxatives, mineral oil, stool softeners, or enemas.

Physical examination

Base your assessment of the patient on the health history information you've collected. Auscultate the abdomen before palpating and percussing. Using this alternative sequence ensures that you don't affect the frequency or intensity of bowel sounds before you assess them.

Inspection. Check the abdomen for distention or scars from previous surgery. Then obtain a baseline measurement of abdominal girth; a later increase may indicate a developing obstruction.

Check his skin temperature and turgor, noting diaphoresis. Then inspect the mucous membranes for signs of dehydration. Note if he has fecal breath odor. Observe his respirations, noting rate and depth. Does he have breathing difficulty or abnormal respiratory patterns?

Auscultation. Next, auscultate the abdomen for bowel sounds. Are they hyperactive, hypoactive, or absent? Then listen for abdominal bruits.

Auscultate the heart, checking the rate and rhythm and noting any abnormal sounds. Also, auscultate the lung fields for crackles and decreased or absent breath sounds. Then, monitor the patient's blood pressure and pulse pressure.

Palpation. As you palpate the abdominal quadrants, note any masses, tenderness, guarding, or rigidity. Palpate the patient's peripheral pulses for rate, rhythm, and intensity.

Percussion. Gently percuss the abdomen to detect pain and abdominal mass.

Life-threatening causes

Your assessment may lead you to suspect one or more of the following.

Complete mechanical intestinal obstruction. The severity and the onset of constipation will vary, depending on the location and extent of the obstruction. With a partial obstruction, constipation may alternate with liquid stool leakage. In a complete obstruction, obstipation may occur.

Constipation can be the earliest sign of a partial colon obstruction, but it usually occurs later when the obstruction is more proximal. The patient may have absent bowel sounds following a period of hyperactive bowel sounds and colicky abdominal pain in the quadrant of the obstruction. This pain may radiate to the flank or lumbar regions. He also may experience abdominal distention and bloating, nausea, and vomiting. Typically, the higher the obstruction, the earlier and more severe the vomiting. In distal small bowel or large bowel obstruction, vomiting is often feculent. In jejunal and duodenal obstruction, nausea and bilious vomiting occur early, and the patient may have an abdominal mass. In the late stages, you'll note a fever, rebound tenderness, and abdominal rigidity. Tachycardia, tachypnea, hypotension and cool, clammy skin indicate shock associated with dehydration and hypovolemia.

The patient may have a history of passing bloody stools. He may also have adhesions from previous abdominal radiation therapy or surgery, or internal or external hernias.

Mesenteric artery infarction. This disorder produces sudden constipation and an inability to expel flatus. Initially, the disorder also produces sudden, colicky, severe midepigastric or periumbilical pain and copious vomiting. Later, the patient may develop abdominal guarding, rigidity, and distention. Bowel sounds disappear after a brief period of hyperactive sounds. You may also auscultate bruits. Accompanying signs of peritonitis, such as fever above 102° F (38.9° C) and abdominal rigidity, signify necrosis.

The patient's history may include an episode of hypoperfusion with a systolic pressure below 90 mm Hg, possibly associated with CHF, dysrhythmias, or hypotension.

Other causes
Certain causes of constipation may not require immediate intervention.

Diagnostic tests. If a patient retains barium administered during a GI study, constipation may occur.

Disorders. Constipation can result from inadequate fluid and fiber intake. It can also stem from neuromuscular disorders that prevent the transmission of nerve impulses to the brain and so decrease the urge to defecate.

Drugs. Constipation may result from narcotic analgesics, such as codeine, hydrocodone, hydromorphone, levorphanol, meperidine, methadone, morphine, oxycodone, oxymorphone, or pentazocine. Other drugs associated with constipation include vinca alkaloids, polystyrene sodium sulfonate, aluminum- or calcium-containing antacids, anticholinergics, and drugs with anticholinergic effects, such as tricyclic antidepressants. Excessive use of laxatives or enemas also causes constipation.

Surgery. Anorectal surgery may traumatize nerves and decrease the urge to defecate, leading to constipation.

Costovertebral angle tenderness

This symptom indicates sudden distention of the renal capsule. Typically, the tenderness is accompanied by dull, constant flank pain in the costovertebral angle (CVA) just lateral to the sacrospinal muscle and below the 12th rib. This associated pain usually travels through the subcostal region toward the umbilicus.

You can elicit CVA tenderness by percussing the CVA. A patient who doesn't have this symptom will feel a thudding, jarring, or pressure-like sensation — but no pain. A patient with CVA tenderness will feel intense pain as the renal capsule stretches, stimulating the afferent nerves that come out of the spinal cord at T11 through L2 to innervate the kidney.

History questions

Explore the patient's problem by asking appropriate questions from this section.

• Find out whether the patient has other symptoms of renal or urologic dysfunction. Ask about his voiding patterns. How often and how much does he usually urinate? Has he noticed any change in fluid intake or output? If so, when did the change occur? Is he experiencing nocturia, dysuria, or tenesmus? Ask about pain or burning during urination. Does he have difficulty starting to urinate? Also ask about the color of his urine. Brown or bright red urine may indicate bleeding.

• Explore other signs and symptoms. Is the patient experiencing any pain in the flank, abdomen, or back? If so, when did he first notice it? How severe is it and where is it? What about nausea and vomiting?

• Determine whether the patient or a family member has a history of urinary tract infection, congenital anomalies, renal calculi, benign prostatic hypertrophy, urinary tract tumors, or other obstructive nephropathies or uropathies. Does the patient have a history of renovascular disorders, such as occlusion of the renal arteries or veins? What about disorders predisposing him to emboli, such as mitral stenosis, infective endocarditis, atrial fibrillation, microthrombi in the left ventricle, rheumatic heart disease, thrombophlebitis of the inferior vena cava or lower legs, congestive heart failure, or recent myocardial infarction?

• Does the patient have a history of disorders that can narrow the arterial lumen, such as periarteritis, blood clots from flank trauma, sickle cell anemia, scleroderma, atherosclerosis, or arteriosclerosis? What about diabetes mellitus, spinal cord injury, or progressive neuromuscular disease? Has he recently undergone urinary catheterization or surgery?

Physical examination

Base your assessment of the patient on the health history information you've collected. When assessing the abdomen, be sure to auscultate before palpating and percussing. This ensures you don't affect the frequency or intensity of bowel sounds before you auscultate them.

Inspection. Examine the patient's skin for signs of trauma, such as hemorrhagic patches around the umbilicus (Cullen's sign) or on the flank (Turner's sign). Note any

ASSESSMENT TIP

Eliciting CVA tenderness

To detect costovertebral angle (CVA) tenderness, have the patient sit upright facing away from you, or have him lie prone. Put the palm of your left hand over his left CVA, then strike the back of your left hand with the ulnar surface of your right fist, as shown. Repeat this percussion technique over the right CVA. A patient with CVA tenderness will experience intense pain.

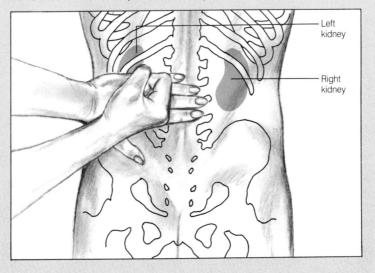

visible swelling or masses in the flank area. Look for autonomic effects of renal pain, such as diaphoresis and pallor, and for signs of shock, such as cool, clammy skin. Inspect the legs for redness and swelling, possibly indicating thrombophlebitis. Also inspect for peripheral edema. Note the color and odor of urine, and monitor for decreased urine output. Observe the patient's respirations, noting rate and depth. Does he have breathing difficulty? Abnormal respiratory pattern?

Auscultation. As you auscultate the abdomen, listen for hypoactive bowel sounds. Auscultate the lungs for crackles, and the heart for tachycardia and any abnormal sounds or murmurs. Then monitor the patient's blood pressure and pulse pressure.

Palpation. Gently palpate over the CVA to assess kidney size. Also, check for abdominal masses. Then palpate the peripheral pulses, noting their rate, rhythm, and intensity.

Percussion. To test for tenderness, percuss the CVA (see *Eliciting CVA tenderness*). Then percuss the abdomen to elicit pain and check for tympanic or dull percussion notes.

Life-threatening causes

Your assessment may lead you to suspect one or more of the following.

Acute pyelonephritis. In this disorder, CVA tenderness occurs with progressive lower abdominal pain that may radiate to the midabdomen or to the groin. The patient may also feel tenderness or pain in the flank area. These characteristic symptoms typically are accompanied by persistent high fever, chills, fatigue, weakness, dysuria, hematuria, nocturia, and urinary urgency, frequency, and tenesmus. The urine may smell like fish or ammonia. Tachycardia, tachypnea, mental confusion, decreased urine output, and hypotension may indicate that bacteremia is progressing to septic shock. Typically, the patient has a history of recent invasive urinary tract procedures, urinary tract obstruction, neurogenic bladder, diabetes, or compromised renal function. Sexually active women are particularly vulnerable. That's because women have a short urethra, which increases the risk of introducing organisms into the urinary tract.

Renal infarction. Usually CVA tenderness will be accompanied by flank pain, severe continuous upper abdominal pain, anorexia, nausea and vomiting, decreased bowel sounds, and fever. You may not be able to palpate the kidneys because of their size. The patient may have a history of a disorder that predisposes him to emboli or narrows the arterial lumen.

Renal trauma. A blunt or penetrating injury to the flank or abdomen may produce CVA tenderness along with flank or abdominal pain that can radiate to the groin. Other findings may include hematuria, oliguria, nausea, vomiting, paralytic ileus, a visible or palpable flank mass, and Turner's sign. Renal laceration or fracture also may produce signs of shock, such as hypotension; tachycardia; narrowed pulse pressure; and cool, clammy skin.

Renal vein occlusion. A rapid onset of thrombosis produces severe lumbar pain as well as CVA and epigastric tenderness. The patient also may experience fever, pallor, hematuria, proteinuria, and peripheral edema. Bilateral obstruction may cause kidney enlargement, oliguria, and possibly hypertension. The patient may have a history of thrombophlebitis of the inferior vena cava or lower legs, congestive heart failure, or periarteritis.

Other causes

CVA tenderness also results from disorders that may not require immediate intervention. Flank pain and CVA tenderness may result from infundibular or ureteropelvic junction calculi. Perirenal abscess also can cause severe CVA tenderness.

Cyanosis

Bluish or bluish black discoloration of the skin and mucous membranes, cyanosis results from an excessive concentration of unoxygenated hemoglobin in the blood. It may develop abruptly or gradually and can be classified as central or peripheral, although the two types may exist together.

Central cyanosis reflects inadequate oxygenation of systemic arterial blood caused by right-to-left cardiac shunting, pulmonary disease, or hematologic disorders. The result is an excessive amount of unsaturated hemoglobin in the arterial blood (SaO_2). You may see central cyanosis anywhere on the skin, the mucous membranes of the mouth and lips, and the conjunctiva.

Peripheral cyanosis reflects sluggish peripheral circulation caused by vasoconstriction, reduced cardiac output, or vascular occlusion. This leads to reduced venous blood oxygen saturation (SvO_2). Peripheral cyanosis may be widespread, or it may occur just in one arm or leg. You won't see peripheral cyanosis on a patient's mucous membranes. Typically, you'll see it on the exposed areas, such as the fingers, nail beds, feet, nose, and ears.

Although cyanosis is an important sign of cardiovascular and pulmonary disorders, it isn't always an accurate gauge of oxygenation. Several factors contribute to its development, including hemoglobin concentration and oxygen saturation, cardiac output, and PaO_2. Usually, cyanosis can be detected only at an unsaturated hemoglobin level of more than 5 g/100 ml of blood. Although severe cyanosis is obvious, mild cyanosis is more difficult to detect — even in natural, bright light. In a dark-skinned patient, mild cyanosis is most apparent in the mucous membranes and nail beds.

Keep in mind that the environment can produce transient non-pathologic cyanosis. Peripheral cyanosis, for example, may result from cutaneous vasoconstriction following brief exposure to cold air or water. Central cyanosis may be caused by reduced PaO_2 at high altitudes.

History questions

Explore the patient's problem by asking appropriate questions from this section.

• How long has the patient had the cyanosis? Does it subside and recur? Does it occur with fatigue or dyspnea? If the cyanosis is peripheral, is it aggravated by cold, smoking, or stress? Is it alleviated by massage or rewarming?

• Does the patient have a cough? Is it productive? If so, have him describe the sputum color and consistency.

• Also ask about associated chest pain. How severe is it? Does it radiate? Does anything aggravate or alleviate it?

• Does he have any pain in his arms and legs — especially when he walks? Any abnormal sensations, such as numbness or tingling, coldness, weakness, or paralysis?

• Review the patient's history, focusing on cardiac, pulmonary, and hematologic disorders. Ask about rheumatic heart disease, myocardial infarction (MI), congestive heart failure (CHF), cardiogenic shock, cardiomyopathy, atherosclerosis, and prosthetic valves. Also ask about asthma, obstructive lung disease, thrombophlebitis, and varicose veins. Has the patient had an acute bleeding episode or septicemia? What about chest, hip, or leg trauma? Find out, too, about recent pregnancy, weight gain, exposure to allergens, or severe emotional stress.

• If the patient's a child, determine whether he's recently experienced a high fever, muffled voice, sore throat, drooling, dysphagia, restlessness, rhinitis, malaise, or anorexia.

• Which medications is the patient taking? Ask about drugs that can precipitate CHF, such as angiotensin converting enzyme inhibitors, antihypertensives, beta blockers, calcium channel blockers, corticosteroids, encainide, nonsteroidal anti-inflammatory drugs, amiodarone, carbamazepine, flecainide, recombinant interferon alfa-2a, or recombinant interleukin-2. Has the patient recently received an ergot injection, an intra-arterial drug injection, or mechanical ventilation under pressure? What about subclavian vein cannulation? Does the patient use aspirin or indomethacin, which could precipitate asthma, or oral contraceptives, which could cause thrombophlebitis?

Physical examination

Base your assessment of the patient on the health history information you've collected.

Inspection. Determine the extent of cyanosis by examining the patient's skin and mucous membranes for coolness, pallor or redness, and ulceration. Note whether the affected arm or leg blanches when elevated even slightly. Also note clubbing, edema, or neck vein distention.

Observe the patient's respirations, noting the rate and depth. Also, note any breathing difficulty or abnormal respiratory patterns. Check for nasal flaring, stridor, audible wheezes, muffled voice, barking cough, costal retractions, and use of accessory muscles. Inspect for asymmetrical chest expansion or barrel chest. Then observe the abdomen for ascites and a visible fluid wave.

Palpation. Check the rate, rhythm, and intensity of peripheral pulses, and test capillary refill time. Palpate the liver for enlargement and tenderness. Then palpate over the lungs to detect decreased vocal or tactile fremitus, decreased diaphragmatic excursion, or subcutaneous crepitation. To evaluate muscle tone and strength, palpate the major muscles.

Percussion. Next, percuss over the liver to detect enlargement and tenderness, and the entire abdomen to detect shifting dullness. Also, percuss over the lungs, noting hyperresonant or tympanic percussion notes.

Auscultation. As you auscultate for heart rate and rhythm, be alert for gallops and murmurs. Also auscultate the abdominal aorta and femoral arteries to detect any bruits. Auscultate the lungs for decreased or adventitious breath sounds, such as wheezes, crackles, or whispered pectoriloquy. Then monitor the patient's blood pressure and pulse pressure.

Life-threatening causes

Your assessment may lead you to suspect one or more of the following.

Asthma. In this disorder, cyanosis is a late sign of hypoxemia resulting from airway obstruction. During an asthma attack, a patient typically experiences dyspnea, tachypnea, intercostal retraction during inspiration and intercostal bulging during expiration, accessory muscle use, and flaring nostrils. During a severe episode, you may note tachycardia, paradoxical pulses, wheezing, or decreased breath sounds. Associated findings may include hyperresonance, decreased vocal and tactile fremitus, and decreased diaphragmatic excursion. The patient may have a history of emotional stress, asthma, or recent exposure to an allergen. Or he may have recently taken aspirin or indomethacin.

Congestive heart failure. Typically, cyanosis is a late sign of CHF. The cyanosis may be central, peripheral, or both. In left ventricular failure, central cyanosis occurs along with tachycardia, fatigue, dyspnea, tachypnea, normal or low blood pressure, cold intolerance, orthopnea, cough, ventricular or atrial gallop, bibasilar crackles, and a diffuse apical impulse. Dependent edema, neck vein distention, and prolonged capillary refill time also may occur. In right ventricular failure, peripheral cyanosis occurs with fatigue, peripheral edema, ascites, jugular vein distention, and hepatomegaly.

Epiglottitis. Cyanosis is a late sign of hypoxemia resulting from airway obstruction by the swollen epiglottis. Earlier signs may include a high fever, muffled voice, sore throat, dysphagia, inspiratory stridor, use of accessory muscles of respiration, decreased breath sounds, tachycardia, anxiety, and drooling. The patient's history may reveal exposure to *Haemophilus influenzae.*

Laryngotracheobronchitis. Cyanosis can occur during a coughing episode associated with acute laryngotracheobronchitis. This harsh, barking cough typically is accompanied by accessory muscle use, restlessness, anxiety, stridor, and tachycardia. Auscultation reveals diminished breath sounds, crackles, and rhonchi. The patient may have a history of rhinitis, fever, malaise, and anorexia for 2 to 3 days before symptoms begin.

Peripheral arterial occlusion (acute). Central cyanosis of one arm or leg or, occasionally, of both legs occurs when the ischemic leg is placed in a dependent position. When ele-vated, the leg blanches. The cyanosis or pallor is accompanied by sharp or aching pain that worsens when the patient moves. Related findings in the affected limb include paresthesia, weakness, paralysis, and pale, cool skin. You may detect decreased or absent peripheral pulses, prolonged capillary refill time (greater than 2 seconds), and bruits over stenotic lesions. The patient's history may include atherosclerosis, dissecting aortic aneurysm, rheumatic heart disease, atrial fibrillation, an intra-arterial drug injection, or ergot-induced vasospasm. He may also have a prosthetic heart valve.

Pneumonia. In this disorder, central cyanosis typically is preceded by fever, shaking chills, and pleuritic chest pain that's exacerbated by deep inspiration. The patient may have a dry or productive cough, depending on the stage and type of pneumonia. Sputum may be discolored and foul-smelling. Associated signs and symptoms can include decreased breath sounds, crackles, wheezing, dullness on percussion, whispered pectoriloquy, tachycardia, tachypnea, myalgia, fatigue, headache, dyspnea, abdominal pain, anorexia, and diaphoresis. The patient's history may include exposure to a contagious organism, hazardous fumes, or air pollution; smoking; or chronic obstructive pulmonary disease (COPD).

Pneumothorax. A cardinal sign of pneumothorax, central cyanosis is accompanied by dyspnea and sudden, sharp, severe chest pain. Often unilateral, this chest pain is rarely localized, and it increases with chest movement. When centrally located and radiating to the neck, the pain may mimic that of an MI. Breath sounds are decreased or absent on the affected side with hyperresonance or tympany, subcutaneous crepitation, and decreased vocal fremitus. Asymmetrical chest expansion, accessory muscle use, nonproductive cough, tachypnea, tachycardia, anxiety, and restlessness also occur. With a tension pneumothorax, you may also observe or palpate tracheal deviation. The patient's health history may reveal recent trauma, subclavian vein cannulation, COPD, lung malignancy, or mechanical ventilation under pressure.

Pulmonary embolism. Central cyanosis occurs when a large embolus obstructs the pulmonary circulation. The cyanosis will be accompanied by the sudden dyspnea that's the hallmark of this disorder and by intense angina-like or pleuritic pain that's aggravated by deep breathing and thoracic movement. Other findings may include anxiety, tachycardia, tachypnea, nonproductive cough or one that produces blood-tinged sputum, low-grade fever, restlessness, diaphoresis, crackles, pleural friction rubs, diffuse wheezing, and dull percussion notes. The patient also may exhibit signs of circulatory collapse (a weak, rapid pulse and hypotension), signs of cerebral ischemia (transient unconsciousness, coma, and seizures), signs of hypoxia (restlessness), and—particularly in elderly patients—hemiplegia and other focal neurologic deficits. Less common signs include massive hemoptysis, chest splinting, leg edema, and distended neck veins. The patient may have a history of thrombophlebitis of the deep systemic veins, varicose veins, hip or leg fractures, acute MI, CHF, cardiogenic shock, congestive

cardiomyopathies, pregnancy, or oral contraceptive use.

Shock. With cardiogenic, hypovolemic, or septic shock, peripheral cyanosis or pallor develops in the hands and feet, which may also be cold and clammy. Related findings include lethargy, confusion, and prolonged capillary refill time (greater than 2 seconds), and a rapid, weak pulse. You may also note tachypnea, hyperpnea, and hypotension. The patient's history may include a disorder predisposing him to shock, such as massive bleeding, left ventricular failure, or septicemia.

Other causes
Cyanosis also results from conditions that may not require immediate intervention.

Disorders. Cyanosis may result from bronchiectasis, Buerger's disease, chronic arteriosclerotic occlusive disease, COPD, congenital heart defects that cause right-to-left intracardiac shunting, cystic fibrosis, deep vein thrombosis, lung cancer, methemoglobinemia, and Raynaud's disease.

Diarrhea

Usually a chief sign of intestinal disorders, diarrhea is an increase in the frequency and fluid content of bowel movements compared with the patient's normal bowel habits. The symptom may be acute or chronic. One or more pathophysiologic mechanisms may contribute to diarrhea (see *Why diarrhea occurs*). The fluid and electrolyte imbalances it produces may precipitate life-

Why diarrhea occurs

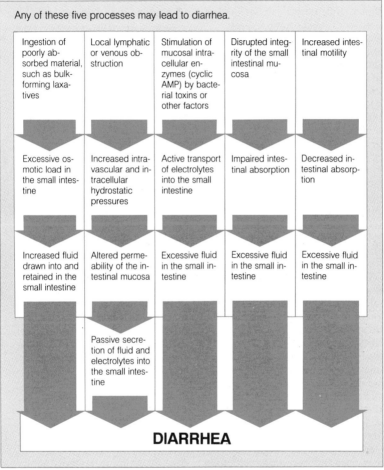

Any of these five processes may lead to diarrhea.

Ingestion of poorly absorbed material, such as bulk-forming laxatives	Local lymphatic or venous obstruction	Stimulation of mucosal intracellular enzymes (cyclic AMP) by bacterial toxins or other factors	Disrupted integrity of the small intestinal mucosa	Increased intestinal motility
Excessive osmotic load in the small intestine	Increased intravascular and intracellular hydrostatic pressures	Active transport of electrolytes into the small intestine	Impaired intestinal absorption	Decreased intestinal absorption
Increased fluid drawn into and retained in the small intestine	Altered permeability of the intestinal mucosa	Excessive fluid in the small intestine	Excessive fluid in the small intestine	Excessive fluid in the small intestine
	Passive secretion of fluid and electrolytes into the small intestine			

DIARRHEA

threatening dysrhythmias or hypovolemic shock.

History questions
Explore the patient's problem by asking appropriate questions from this section.
• Ask the patient when he started passing diarrheal stools, and have him describe their frequency and character. Has he had similar episodes of diarrhea before?
• Also ask about any associated abdominal pain or cramping. Is the pain constant, or does it alternate with pain-free periods? When did the pain begin and where is it? Is he experiencing nausea and

vomiting? If so, have him describe the color and odor of the vomitus.
• What about other signs and symptoms, such as anorexia, weakness, fatigue, exertional dyspnea, palpitations, muscle tremors, and confusion? If appropriate, ask a female patient if she's experienced decreased or absent menses. Ask a family member if he's noticed any changes in the patient's personality.
• Have the patient describe a typical day's menu, and note whether his intake of fruit or fiber is excessive. Has he changed his diet recently? Does he have any known food allergies or a lactase deficiency? Has he been under unusual stress lately?
• Determine whether the patient has a history of GI disorders, such as ulcerative colitis or Crohn's disease; thyroid disorders; or exposure to bacterial or viral gastroenteritis. Has he had a recent episode of hypoperfusion, such as congestive heart failure (CHF), severe hypotension, or cardiac dysrhythmias? What about surgery or radiation therapy?
• Find out what medications the patient's taking. Antibiotics may cause pseudomembranous enterocolitis. Is he taking anything to treat his diarrhea? How often does he use laxatives?

Physical examination

Base your assessment of the patient on the health history information you've collected. When assessing the abdomen, be sure to auscultate before palpating and percussing. This alternative sequence ensures that you don't affect the frequency and intensity of bowel sounds before you auscultate them.

Inspection. Examine the patient's skin and oral mucosa, noting color, temperature, and turgor. Then inspect his nails for pulsations in the capillary beds. As you observe his abdomen, note any distention, visible peristaltic waves, or bulging intestinal loops.

Inspect for exophthalmos. Next, observe the patient's respirations, noting the rate and depth. Also, note any breathing difficulty and abnormal respiratory patterns. Observe the patient's level of consciousness and emotional state.

Be sure to record the color, odor, and consistency of any diarrhea or vomitus.

Auscultation. Next, auscultate the abdominal quadrants for bowel sounds and characterize their quality. Also, listen to the lungs for abnormal sounds, particularly crackles and rhonchi. Monitor the patient's blood pressure and pulse pressure.

Palpation. As you palpate the abdomen, note any rigidity, guarding, or tenderness. Also palpate peripheral pulses for rate, rhythm, and intensity. Carefully palpate the neck for thyroid gland enlargement.

Percussion. Gently percuss the abdomen. You'll hear tympany over gas pockets and dullness over fluid-filled areas.

Life-threatening causes

Your assessment may lead you to suspect one or more of the following.

Intestinal obstruction (partial). Intermittent diarrhea and constipation may accompany short episodes of intense, colicky, cramping pain that alternate with pain-free periods. Related findings may include abdominal distention, tenderness, and guarding; tympanic percussion notes; visible peristaltic waves; and pain-induced agitation. On auscultation, you'll hear high-pitched, tinkling, or hyperactive bowel sounds proximal to the obstruction and lower-pitched, hypoactive, or absent bowel sounds distally. In jejunal and duodenal obstruction, nausea and bilious vomiting occur early; in distal small-bowel or large-bowel obstruction, nausea and vomiting are often feculent. If the patient goes into hypovolemic shock, you'll detect hypotension, tachycardia, tachypnea, and cool, clammy skin. The patient may have adhesions from previous abdominal radiation therapy or surgery. He also may have passed blood-tinged stools.

Mesenteric artery ischemia. In this disorder, bloody diarrhea alternating with constipation occurs with severe, constant, and diffuse abdominal pain. Typically, the diarrhea is preceded by 2 to 3 days of colicky periumbilical pain. Associated findings include vomiting, anorexia, and, in the late stages, extreme abdominal tenderness with rigidity. Hypotension, tachycardia, tachypnea, and cool, clammy skin indicate hypovolemic or septic shock. The patient's history may include a recent episode of hypoperfusion, such as CHF, cardiac dysrhythmias, hypotension, or shock.

Pseudomembranous enterocolitis. This disorder produces copious amounts of extremely watery, mucoid diarrhea that develops suddenly and rapidly precipitates shock. Other indications include colicky abdominal pain and disten-tion, fever, nausea, vomiting, signs of dehydration, and disorienta-tion. Typically, the health history

includes major abdominal surgery or an extended use of broad-spectrum antibiotics, particularly with an elderly or debilitated patient.

Thyrotoxicosis (thyroid storm). Diarrhea, often resulting in dehy-dration, occurs with a sudden rise in systolic pressure, widened pulse pressure, tachycardia, bounding pulse, pulsations in the capillary nail beds, and palpitations. Other physical findings include exopthal-mos; an enlarged thyroid; warm, moist skin; heat intolerance; exer-tional dyspnea; and a temperature over 100° F (37.8° C). Nervousness and emotional lability also occur, with occasional outbursts or, possibly, psychotic behavior. A patient with latent hyperthyroidism may have a history of excessive iodine intake and repeated episodes of symptoms following stressful conditions, such as surgery, infec-tions, pregnancy, or diabetic ketoacidosis. A female patient may have a history of decreased or absent menses.

Other causes
Certain causes of diarrhea may not signal the need for immediate intervention.

Disorders. Diarrhea occurs in bacterial, viral or protozoal gas-troenteritis; carcinoid syndrome; Crohn's disease; irritable bowel syndrome; large bowel neoplasms; lead poisoning; malabsorption syndrome; and ulcerative colitis. It also can stem from food allergy, lactase deficiency, or excessive intake of fruit or fiber.

Drugs. Many drugs can produce diarrhea. The list includes anabolic steroids, androgens, antibiotics (cephalosporins, penicillins, tetracyclines, and clindamycin, erythromycin, lincomycin), cholinergics, estrogens, oral contraceptives, and thyroid hormones. Other drugs that can produce diarrhea include acetohydroxamic acid, auranofin, azacytidine, bentiromide, chenodiol, cisplatin, clofibrate, colchicine, dantrolene, dehydrocholic acid, dicumarol, digitalis, emetine, ethacrynic acid, ethotoin, floxuridine, flucytosine, flutamide, fenfluramine, gemfibrozil, guanethidine, hydroxyurea, indomethacin, ketoprofen, lactulose, l-carnitine, lisinopril, magnesium-containing antacids, mecamylamine, meclofenamate, mefenamic acid, methotrexate, metyrosine, oxyphenbutazone, pancreatin, phentolamine, phenylbutazone, probucol, procainamide, quinacrine, quinidine, sodium polystyrene sulfonate, tolazoline, and trilostane. Laxative abuse can also cause acute or chronic diarrhea.

Surgery. Diarrhea can result from GI tract surgery such as gastrectomy, gastroenterostomy, and pyloroplasty.

Treatment. High-dose radiation therapy can lead to diarrhea.

Dyspnea

Dyspnea is the sensation of difficult or uncomfortable breathing. Typically, a patient calls this symptom shortness of breath. Its severity, which varies greatly, is often unrelated to the severity of the underlying cause. Dyspnea may arise suddenly or slowly and may subside rapidly or persist for years. Depending on the cause of dyspnea, emergency intervention may be necessary (see *Case in point: When dyspnea denotes distress*).

Most people experience dyspnea from overexertion, the severity depending on their physical condition. In a healthy person, rest quickly relieves dyspnea.

History questions

Explore the patient's problem by asking appropriate questions from this section. If he needs emergency care, ask the questions as you intervene.

• Did the shortness of breath begin suddenly or gradually? Is it constant or intermittent? Does it occur during activity or while the patient is resting? Do the attacks awaken the patient at night?

• Has the patient had dyspneic attacks before? If so, is this episode similar or more severe? Does he know what precipitates and alleviates the attacks?

• Does he also have a productive or nonproductive cough or chest pain? What about nausea, vomiting, or diaphoresis? Also ask about dizziness, light-headedness, weakness, fatigue, palpitations, or cold intolerance?

• Has the patient recently experienced trauma or emotional stress? Has he aspirated a foreign body or been exposed to an allergen, contagious organism, fire, steam, superheated air, or fumes from burning chemicals or synthetic materials? Has he recently undergone cardiopulmonary resuscitation, subclavian cannulation, or mechanical ventilation under pressure?

• If the patient is a child, find out if he's recently experienced a sore throat, anorexia, rhinitis, difficulty eating, barking cough, noisy respirations, or fever.

• Does the patient have a history of upper respiratory tract infections,

Case in point: When dyspnea denotes distress

When you suspect an emergency, you need to perform a quick but thorough assessment to determine if the patient's primary symptom truly signals a real danger. That way, you'll be in a position to intervene effectively, if needed.

To help you respond appropriately to a suspected emergency, suppose you're caring for John Peterson, age 42, who suffers a cardiac arrest while at home. Mr. Peterson's wife immediately starts cardiopulmonary resuscitation (CPR) while his daughter rushes to call an ambulance. When the paramedics arrive, they attach a cardiac monitor, which indicates ventricular tachycardia. So they use defibrillation, and after consulting with the doctor at the emergency department (ED), start administering lidocaine. Then, they take Mr. Peterson to the ED.

Once he's stable, he's transferred to your unit for further treatment and monitoring.

Assess first
On your unit, you notice that Mr. Peterson is having trouble breathing. He tells you that it hurts to breathe, particularly on his left side. When you inspect his chest, you find asymmetrical chest wall expansion and accessory muscle use during respirations. You notice that he's restless and tachypneic, and he's getting extremely anxious.

You palpate his chest and find subcutaneous crepitation and evidence of a rib fracture on his left side. When you palpate his neck, you discover that his trachea is deviated. You can't hear any breath sounds on the left side.

Interpret findings and intervene
Your assessment findings lead you to believe that Mr. Peterson may have a tension pneumothorax – a serious complication of CPR. So you immediately call the doctor. You ask another nurse to help set up the equipment needed to insert a chest tube and start underwater seal drainage. Mr. Peterson is already receiving oxygen at the rate of 2 to 4 liters/minute by nasal cannula.

While waiting for the doctor, you help Mr. Peterson into the high Fowler's position, which allows his unaffected lung to expand as much as possible. You keep a careful eye on Mr. Peterson, assessing the rate and depth of his respirations. You also observe him for any breathing difficulty. Then you monitor his level of consciousness, a sensitive indicator of adequate tissue oxygenation.

When the doctor arrives, you help him insert a chest tube, which will remove air from Mr. Peterson's pleural cavity. After the tube is inserted, Mr. Peterson's breathing improves dramatically.

You continue monitoring Mr. Peterson's respiratory status, making sure the underwater seal drainage system is patent and working properly. You note fluctuation and intermittent bubbling in the water seal chamber. You also check for signs of complications, such as increasing dyspnea, air hunger, nasal flaring, subcutaneous emphysema, distended neck veins, hypotension, and tracheal deviation.

Evaluate your care
By performing a quick but systematic assessment of Mr. Peterson, you determined that his main symptom signaled real danger. When you recognized that his other signs and symptoms indicated a tension pneumothorax, you alerted the doctor and began immediate life-saving treatment.

asthma, or chronic obstructive pulmonary disease? Also ask about deep vein thrombophlebitis, varicose veins, cardiac disease, hip or leg fractures, or a recent pregnancy.
• Find out what medications the patient is taking, if any, and ask about any known drug allergies. Is he taking aspirin, indomethacin, or oral contraceptives? What about drugs that can precipitate cardiac dysrhythmias, congestive heart failure (CHF), or myocardial infarction (MI)? Also ask about drugs, such as aspirin, penicillins and other antibiotics, and beta blockers, that can cause bronchoconstriction in sensitive persons.

Physical examination
Base your assessment of the patient on the health history information you've collected.

Inspection. Observe the patient's respirations, noting rate and depth. Look too for difficult breathing and abnormal respiratory patterns. Also, check for grunting respirations, pursed-lip expirations, intercostal retractions during inspiration and bulging during expiration, flaring nostrils, inspiratory stridor, and in children, muffled voice. Look for signs of chronic dyspnea, such as accessory muscle hypertrophy — especially in the shoulders and neck.

Also, observe the patient for peripheral edema, clubbing of the fingers, barrel chest, distended neck veins, and diaphoresis. Inspect for oropharyngeal edema, singed nasal hairs, orofacial burns, prolonged capillary refill time, chest bruising, ascites, and cool, clammy skin. Note the color, consistency, and odor of any sputum.

Palpation. Gently palpate the neck for tracheal deviation and the abdomen for hepatomegaly. Then palpate the chest for asymmetrical chest expansion, decreased diaphragmatic excursion, subcutaneous crepitation, and decreased vocal and tactile fremitus. Also check the patient's peripheral pulses, noting their rate, rhythm, and intensity.

Percussion. Next, percuss over both lungs, noting hyperresonant, dull, or tympanic percussion notes.

Auscultation. Check the lungs for crackles, rhonchi, wheezing, decreased or absent unilateral breath sounds, egophony, bronchophony, whispered pectoriloquy, and pleural friction rubs. Auscultate the heart for tachycardia, pericardial friction rubs, and abnormal sounds or rhythms, such as ventricular or atrial gallop. Finally, monitor blood pressure and pulse pressure.

Life-threatening causes
Your assessment may lead you to suspect one or more of the following.

Adult respiratory distress syndrome (ARDS). Usually, a patient with this progressive respiratory disorder first complains of acute dyspnea and tachypnea. He then develops anxiety, restlessness, decreased mental acuity, grunting respirations, accessory muscle use, tachycardia, crackles, wheezes, rhonchi and, in late stages, cyanosis. Severe ARDS can produce signs of shock, such as hypotension and cool, clammy skin. Typically, the patient has no history of underlying cardiac or pulmonary disease but has sustained a recent pulmonary or systemic insult. (For more information, see *What causes ARDS?*)

Airway obstruction (partial). Acute dyspnea and inspiratory stridor occur as the patient tries to overcome the obstruction. Related findings may include accessory muscle use, tachypnea, decreased or unilateral absent breath sounds, asymmetrical chest expansion, anxiety, cyanosis, diaphoresis, and hypotension. The patient may have aspirated vomitus or a foreign body or been exposed to an allergen. He also may have a disorder that causes copious mouth secretions.

Asthma. Acute dyspneic attacks occur in this chronic disorder, along with dry cough, accessory muscle use, nasal flaring, intercostal and supraclavicular retractions, tachypnea, tachycardia, diaphoresis, prolonged expiration, flushing or cyanosis, and apprehension. On auscultation, you'll note wheezing and rhonchi or decreased breath sounds during a severe episode. On palpation, you'll detect decreased vocal and tactile fremitus and decreased diaphragmatic excursion. Hyperresonance occurs on chest percussion. You may find the patient has a history of asthma or recent exposure to an allergen, emotional stress, or ingestion of aspirin or indomethacin.

Cardiac dysrhythmias. In some dysrhythmias, acute or gradual dyspnea can result from decreased cardiac output. The dyspnea may be accompanied by pulsus alternans, dizziness, light-headedness, weakness, fatigue, and palpitations. Auscultation typically reveals a heart rate greater than 100 beats/minute or less than 60 beats/minute, or an irregular rhythm. The patient may have a history of previous cardiac disease. Or he may be taking medications that can cause dysrhythmias—cardiac glycosides or certain beta blockers, for example.

What causes ARDS?

Dyspnea is a characteristic sign in various conditions that may lead to adult respiratory distress syndrome (ARDS). The following list includes the most common underlying causes:

- aspiration of gastric contents
- drug ingestion and overdose
- hydrocarbon ingestion
- trauma and hemorrhagic shock
- near-drowning
- smoke or gas inhalation
- disseminated intravascular coagulation
- septic shock
- fat and air embolism
- severe pneumonitis (viral and other)
- oxygen toxicity
- postperfusion (cardiopulmonary bypass)
- anaphylaxis
- uremia
- hemorrhagic pancreatitis
- head injury
- homologous blood transfusion.

Congestive heart failure. In this disorder, dyspnea usually develops gradually or occurs as chronic paroxysmal nocturnal dyspnea. In left ventricular failure, dyspnea occurs with tachycardia, fatigue, tachypnea, normal or low blood pressure, cold intolerance, orthopnea, cough, central cyanosis, ventricular or atrial gallop, bibasilar crackles, and diffuse apical impulse. You may also note dependent edema, neck vein distention, and prolonged capillary refill time (greater than 2 seconds). In right ventricular failure, dyspnea occurs with fatigue, peripheral edema, ascites, jugular vein distention, peripheral cyanosis, and hepatomegaly. The patient may have a history of cardiovascular disease, dyspneic episodes, fatigue, weight gain, pallor or cyanosis, diaphoresis, or anxiety. His medication history may include drugs that can precipitate CHF, such as amiodarone, certain beta blockers, or corticosteroids.

Epiglottitis. Dyspnea may occur with inspiratory stridor, accessory muscle use, tachycardia, decreased breath sounds, high fever, muffled voice, sore throat, anxiety, drooling, or dysphagia. Cyanosis is a late sign of hypoxemia resulting from airway obstruction of the swollen epiglottis. The patient's history may include exposure to the organism *Haemophilus influenzae*.

Flail chest. In this disorder, sudden dyspnea results from multiple rib fractures. You'll also see paradoxical chest movements, severe chest pain, hypotension, tachypnea, tachycardia, and cyanosis. On the affected side, you note bruising and decreased or absent breath sounds. The patient will have blunt chest trauma, perhaps from cardiopulmonary resuscitation.

Inhalation injury. Dyspnea may develop suddenly or gradually over several hours after inhalation of chemicals or hot gases. Increasing hoarseness, persistent cough, sooty or bloody sputum, and oropharyngeal edema may occur. Related findings may include thermal burns, singed nasal hairs, and orofacial burns, along with crackles, rhonchi, and wheezes. Signs of respiratory distress may develop. The patient's history will include inhalation of steam, superheated air, smoke from a fire, or fumes from burning chemicals or synthetic materials.

Laryngotracheobronchitis. Dyspnea can occur during a coughing episode associated with acute laryngotracheobronchitis. Associated findings include a harsh and barking cough, accessory muscle use, restlessness, anxiety, stridor, and tachycardia. On auscultation, you'll note diminished breath sounds, crackles, and rhonchi. The patient may have a history of rhinitis, fever, malaise, and anorexia for 2 to 3 days before the onset of symptoms.

Myocardial infarction. In MI, sudden dyspnea occurs with crushing substernal chest pain that may radiate to the back, neck, jaw, and arms. Other signs and symptoms include nausea, vomiting, diaphoresis, vertigo, hypertension or hypotension, tachycardia, anxiety, and pale, cool, clammy skin. Patient history findings may include heart disease, hypertension, hypercholesterolemia, or use of drugs that can precipitate an MI—for example cocaine, dextrothyroxine, estramustine phosphate sodium, or recombinant interleukin-2.

Pneumonia. Dyspnea occurs suddenly, usually accompanied by fever, shaking chills, and pleuritic chest pain that worsens with deep inspiration. The patient also will have a dry or productive cough, depending on the stage and type of pneumonia; any sputum may be discolored and foul-smelling. Associated signs and symptoms may include decreased breath sounds, crackles, rhonchi, dullness on percussion, whispered pectoriloquy, tachycardia, tachypnea, myalgia, fatigue, headache, abdominal pain, anorexia, central cyanosis, and diaphoresis. His history may include exposure to a contagious organism, hazardous fumes, or air pollution; smoking; or chronic obstructive pulmonary disease (COPD).

Pneumothorax. Acute dyspnea and central cyanosis occur with sudden, severe, sharp chest pain. This pain is often unilateral, rarely localized, and increases with chest movement. On the affected side, breath sounds are decreased or absent. You'll also note hyperresonance or tympany, subcutaneous crepitation, and decreased vocal fremitus. Related findings include asymmetrical chest expansion, accessory muscle use, a nonproductive cough, tachypnea, tachycardia, anxiety, and restlessness. With tension pneumothorax, tracheal deviation also occurs. The patient's history may include recent subclavian vein cannulation, COPD, lung malignancy, or mechanical ventilation under pressure.

Pulmonary edema. Severe dyspnea will often be preceded by signs of CHF, such as distended neck veins and orthopnea. Other findings include tachycardia, tachypnea, crackles in both lung fields, S_3 gallop, oliguria, thready pulse, hypotension, diaphoresis, cyanosis, and marked anxiety. The patient's cough may be dry or produce copious amounts of pink, frothy sputum. His health history may reveal cardiovascular disease, dyspnea, fatigue, weight gain, pallor or cyanosis, diaphoresis, or anxiety.

Pulmonary embolism. The sudden dyspnea that's the hallmark of this disorder occurs along with intense angina-like or pleuritic pain aggravated by deep breathing and thoracic movement. Central cyanosis occurs when a large embolus obstructs pulmonary circulation. Other findings may include anxiety, tachycardia, tachypnea, a nonproductive cough or one that produces blood-tinged sputum, low-grade fever, restlessness, diaphoresis, crackles, pleural friction rubs, diffuse wheezing, and dull percussion notes. You may also note signs of circulatory collapse, signs of cerebral ischemia, signs of hypoxia, and—particularly in elderly patients—hemiplegia and other focal neurologic deficits. The patient's history may include thrombophlebitis of the deep systemic veins, varicose veins, hip or leg fractures, acute MI, CHF, cardiogenic shock, congestive cardiomyopathy, pregnancy or oral contraceptive use.

Other causes
Certain causes of dyspnea may not signal the need for immediate intervention.

Disorders. Dyspnea occurs in amyotrophic lateral sclerosis (Lou Gehrig's disease), anemia, severe anxiety, cor pulmonale, emphysema, Guillain-Barré syndrome, interstitial lung cancer, pleural effusion, poliomyelitis (bulbar), and tuberculosis.

Drugs. Dyspnea is an adverse effect of bitolterol, dopamine, encainide, epinephrine, ergot alkaloids, muromonab-CD3, nitroprusside, NSAIDs, and interferons. It can result from a disulfiram reaction. It also can result from the use of beta blockers, cholinergics, neuromuscular blockers, acetylcysteine, dinoprostone, flecainide, and vindesine, which can cause bronchospasm; and amiodarone, busulfan, melphalan, and mephenytoin, which can cause pulmonary fibrosis. Drugs that produce a hypersensitivity reaction, particularly quinidine, penicillins, cephalosporins, and salicylates, can cause dyspnea associated with asthma or laryngospasm. Withdrawal from corticosteroid therapy also may cause dyspnea.

Fontanel bulging

In a normal infant, the anterior fontanel (soft spot) is flat and soft but firm, and can be clearly distinguished from the surrounding skull bones. It may show subtle pulsations, reflecting the pulse. (See *Locating the fontanels*).

A bulging fontanel — one that's widened and tense, and shows marked pulsations — is a cardinal sign of increased intracranial pressure (ICP), a potentially life-threatening emergency.

History questions
Explore the patient's problem by asking the parents appropriate questions from this section.
• When did you first notice the bulging? Has it been getting worse?
• Has the infant's behavior changed? Has he vomited frequently, lost interest in feeding, or appeared lethargic? Have the parents noted high-pitched crying?
• Is the infant on (or has he recently been on) a mechanical ventilator? Has he recently had an infection? What about head trauma, including birth trauma?
• Ask if the infant or any family member has had a recent rash or

Locating the fontanels

The anterior fontanel lies at the junction of the sagittal, coronal, and frontal sutures. Normally, it measures about 1″ (2.5 cm) by 1½″ to 2″ (4 to 5 cm) at birth. By age 20 months, the anterior fontanel usually closes.

The posterior fontanel lies at the junction of the sagittal and lambdoid sutures. If it hasn't already fused by the time of birth, it measures ⅜″ to ¾″ (1 to 2 cm) and usually closes by age 2 months.

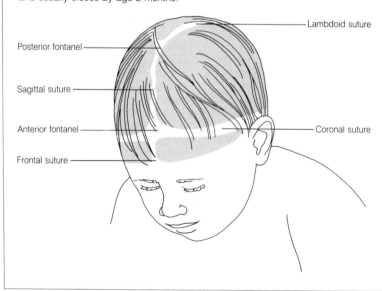

Lambdoid suture
Posterior fontanel
Sagittal suture
Anterior fontanel
Frontal suture
Coronal suture

fever. Does he have a brain tumor or hydrocephalus?

Physical examination

Base your assessment of the patient on the health history information you've collected.

Inspection. Transient physiologic bulging may result when an infant lies down for a prolonged period, coughs, or cries. Therefore, you should observe the patient's head while he's upright and relaxed to determine if the bulging is abnormal. After noting the overall shape of the patient's head, measure its circumference and the size of the fontanel. Look for distended scalp veins.

Assess the infant's level of consciousness by observing spontaneous activity, postural reflex activity, and sensory responses. Does he assume a normal flexed posture or one of extreme extension, opisthotonos, or hypotonia? Observe how he moves his arms and legs; excessive tremors or frequent twitching may signal the onset of a seizure.

Inspect the patient's eyes. Are they deviated downward? Then check pupillary response to light. Is it decreased or absent? Look, too, for other signs of increased ICP, such as abnormal breathing patterns and a distinctive, high-pitched cry. Check the rate and depth of the infant's respirations. Is he having difficulty breathing?

Palpation. As you palpate the fontanel, be sure the infant is upright to avoid any transient physiologic bulging. Note any fullness or tension. Then check the muscles for flaccidity. Palpate the peripheral pulses, noting their rate, rhythm, and intensity.

Percussion. Check the infant's reflexes for abnormal responses.

Auscultation. Neurogenic pulmonary edema can develop in children with increased ICP, so auscultate the lungs for adventitious sounds, particularly crackles. Auscultate, too, for abnormal heart sounds or rate. Monitor the patient's blood pressure and pulse pressure.

Life-threatening cause

Your assessment may lead you to suspect this disorder.

Increased ICP. A full, tense, bulging fontanel and increased head circumference are early signs of increased ICP in an infant. Other signs and symptoms are often subtle and difficult to discern. They may include behavioral changes, such as irritability that increases when the infant's head is moved, lethargy, disinterest in feeding, and vomiting. The infant may show an abnormal respiratory pattern such as Cheyne-Stokes respirations, central neurogenic hyperventilation, or apneustic, ataxic, or cluster breathing. He may also have a distinctive, high-pitched cry. Scalp veins may be distended, and the eyes may be deviated downward — known as sunset eyes.

As ICP rises, the spaces between the cranial bones may become palpable, the pupils may dilate, and the patient may become drowsy and eventually slip into a coma. Seizures commonly develop. In the late stages, you may note tachycardia and fluctuating blood pressure progressing to hypotension. You may also observe decorticate, decerebrate, or other abnormal posturing. The infant's history may include prematurity with respiratory distress syndrome, use of mechanical ventilation, head trauma, hydro-cephalus, or brain tumor.

Headache

The most common neurologic symptom, headache may be mild to severe, localized or generalized, constant or intermittent, throbbing or viselike. About 90% of all headaches result from vascular causes, tension, or a combination of the two. (The vascular causes are more common in women than in men.) Headaches may also result from sinus or ocular problems or from metabolic conditions, such as hyperglycemia.

Occasionally, headache results from inflammation or increased pressure in the cranium. In such cases, it indicates a severe neurologic disorder that requires immediate attention. (For more information, see *What causes headache?*)

PATHOPHYSIOLOGY

What causes headache?

Headache pain can be intracranial or extracranial. Like other types of pain, headache depends on stimulation of specialized pain receptors. However, most cranial structures, including the brain parenchyma, choroid plexus, pia arachnoid membrane, parts of the dura mater, ventricular linings, and the skull itself, don't contain pain receptors. Intracranial structures responsive to pain include the blood vessels, venous sinuses and their tributaries, sensory cranial nerves, dural arteries, and the arteries and dura at the base of the brain. Extracranial structures sensitive to pain include the skin, scalp, and mucosa.

Extracranial pain
Three cranial nerves transmit pain sensations. The trigeminal (V) nerve contains the pain fibers above the tentorium cerebelli; pain is referred to the frontal and temporal areas as far back as above the ears. The glossopharyngeal (IX) and vagus (X) nerves contain the pain fibers for structures below the tentorium cerebelli. Usually, these nerves transmit pain impulses from the occipital and upper cervical areas.

Pain stemming from the sinuses, ears, eyes, or teeth results from inflammation of the ostia or turbinates or from displacement of the cranial nerves, causing referred pain to the head.

Intracranial pain
The pain of meningitis is thought to be caused by a chemical irritation of the meningeal nerve endings (see illustration). Ruptured cerebral aneurysm, acute epidural hemorrhage, intracerebral hemorrhage, subarachnoid hemorrhage, and subdural hematoma all stimulate meningeal nerve endings, causing a chemical meningitis.

Space-occupying lesions and enlargement of brain tissue—which occurs with brain abscess, brain tumor, hematoma, or brain edema—cause headache by displacing pain-sensitive structures (see illustration). Dilation of the cranial arteries by such disorders as hypertension, acute cerebrovascular insufficiency, hypercapnia, hypoxia, or toxic systemic reactions, as well as the use of vasodilators, also cause headache by displacement of these pain-sensitive structures.

History questions
Explore the patient's problem by asking appropriate questions from this section.
• Have the patient describe his headache. Exactly where is the pain? How intense is it? Ask him to characterize the pain. For instance, is it dull, throbbing, or knifelike?
• How long has the patient had the headache? Has it changed in any way since it began? If so, how? Does he recall experiencing any prodromal symptoms? Does anything exacerbate the pain?
• If the patient is an infant, ask the parents if he's behaved as if he has a headache—perhaps by banging or holding his head.
• Find out if the patient has any associated signs or symptoms, such as fever, nausea, vomiting, stiff neck, weakness, decreased pain perception and sensation in the limbs, drowsiness, confusion, eye pain, photophobia, visual disturbances, or dizziness.
• Has the patient ever had a similar

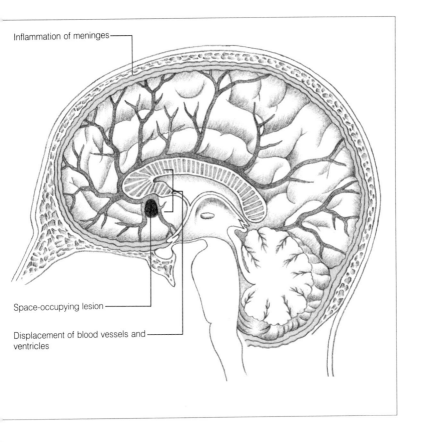

Inflammation of meninges

Space-occupying lesion

Displacement of blood vessels and ventricles

headache? If so, how often does he get such headaches and how long do they usually last?

• Ask family members if they've noticed severe muscle twitching, speaking or walking difficulties, seizures, or changes in the patient's personality or level of consciousness (LOC).

• Check for any precipitating factors. Has the patient been under an unusual amount of stress? Has he recently experienced head trauma, dental work, or sinus, ear, or systemic infections? If he's experienced head trauma, find out when and how it occurred. Has he been exposed to any organisms that commonly cause meningitis or encephalitis?

• If the patient is a school-age child, ask the parents about his recent school performance and any problems at home that may be a source of tension. If the patient is an adult, have him describe his work environment, including lighting, temperature, noise level, and the like. Ask if he uses a video display terminal.

• Ask if the patient has a history of smoking, cardiovascular disease, hypertension, blood dyscrasias, hemorrhagic disorders, seizures, glaucoma, or poor vision.

• Ask about medications the patient may be taking. Indomethacin, digoxin, aspirin, and anticoagulants such as coumadin can cause headache.

Physical examination

Base your assessment of the patient on the health history information you've collected.

Inspection. Observe the rate and depth of the patient's respirations. See if he's having difficulty breathing, and check for any abnormal patterns. Then examine his head for bruises, bleeding, swelling, and erythema of the sinus areas, as well as for other signs of trauma. Check for neck stiffness, otorrhea, rhinorrhea, or Battle's sign.

Next, assess the patient's LOC. Is he restless, drowsy, lethargic, stuporous, or comatose? Check his eyes, noting pupillary size, equality, and reaction to light. Also, look for downward or conjugate deviation, photophobia, redness over the eye, a cloudy cornea, a hardened eyeball, swelling, or ptosis.

Check for tremors when the patient is resting and when he's performing an intentional activity. Is his motor ability symmetrical? Does he assume any abnormal positions, such as opisthotonos or decerebrate or decorticate posture? If he's alert, you can check for cranial nerve involvement by having him smile widely and raise his eyebrows.

If the patient is an infant, inspect the fontanels for bulging. Note the child's behavior. Is he banging or holding his head? If he's crying, is the cry high-pitched or shrill?

Palpation. Gently palpate the scalp for tenderness and crepitus and palpate the sinuses for tender, painful spots. If head trauma has been ruled out, slowly move the neck through a small range of motion to check for pain or nuchal rigidity. Assess the patient's motor strength by having him squeeze your hands. Note any inequality in his grip. As you palpate peripheral pulses, note their rate, rhythm, and intensity.

Percussion. Gently percuss the lung fields, listening for any abnormal dullness or hyperresonance. Check the patient for a positive Babinski's reflex. As you percuss his reflexes, note any hyperreflexia.

Auscultation. As you auscultate over the temporal artery, listen for bruits. Auscultate all lung fields for adventitious breath sounds, especially crackles and rhonchi. When you auscultate the heart, listen for abnormal sounds such as S_3 — an indicator of left ventricular failure. Monitor the patient's blood pressure and pulse pressure.

Life- and vision-threatening causes

Your assessment may lead you to suspect one or more of the following.

Brain abscess. A headache stemming from this cause typically intensifies over a few days, localizes to a particular spot, and is aggravated by straining. The headache may be accompanied by nausea, vomiting, and focal or generalized seizures. The patient's LOC varies from drowsiness to deep stupor. Depending on the abscess site, associated signs and symptoms may include aphasia, impaired visual acuity, hemiparesis, ataxia, tremor, and personality changes. Signs of infection, such as fever and pallor, usually develop late, if at all. In one out of two cases, the abscess remains encapsulated and isn't likely to produce such signs. The patient may have a history of systemic, chronic middle ear, mastoid, or sinus infection; compound fracture or osteomyelitis of the skull; or a penetrating head wound.

Cerebral aneurysm (ruptured). In this disorder, a sudden, excruciating, (sometimes unilateral) headache develops, usually peaking within minutes. Most often, the headache is quickly followed by loss of consciousness or an altered LOC. Depending on the severity and location of the bleeding, the patient may also have nausea and vomiting, ataxia, hemiparesis, hemisensory deficit, downward or conjugate deviation of the eye toward the side of the lesion, and miotic but reactive pupils. You may also note signs and symptoms of meningeal irritation, such as nuchal rigidity and blurred vision. The patient's history may include hypertension or other cardiovascular disorders, a stressful life-style, or smoking.

Encephalitis. A patient with this disorder will have a severe, generalized headache accompanied by a deteriorating LOC over 48 hours — perhaps from lethargy to coma. Associated signs and symptoms include fever, nuchal rigidity, irritability, seizures, nausea, vomiting, photophobia, focal neurologic deficits such as hemiparesis and hemiplegia, and cranial nerve palsies such as ptosis. The patient may have a history of exposure to viruses that commonly cause encephalitis, such as arboviruses, mumps virus, or herpes simplex viruses.

Epidural hemorrhage (acute). A progressively severe headache will immediately follow a brief loss of consciousness and a rapid, steady decline in LOC. The headache is often accompanied by nausea and vomiting, unilateral seizures, contralateral hemiparesis, hemiplegia, high fever, ipsilateral pupil dilation, and signs of increasing intracranial pressure (ICP). The patient's history will probably reveal head trauma within the last 24 hours.

Glaucoma (acute closed-angle). This disorder endangers the patient's sight. The severe eye pain that can signal an acute glaucoma episode is often accompanied by headache. Associated signs and symptoms include blurred vision, halo vision, redness over the affected eye, photophobia, a cloudy cornea, a hardened eyeball, a swollen upper eyelid, and a moderately dilated, fixed pupil. The increased intraocular pressure may also produce nausea and vomiting. The patient may have a history of chronic glaucoma, elevated intraocular pressure, or increasingly blurred vision.

Intracerebral hemorrhage (acute).
With this disorder, a severe, generalized headache may start suddenly or gradually. The patient may also experience decreased LOC — commonly progressing to coma — hypertension, and, occasionally, nuchal rigidity and vomiting. Other signs and symptoms vary with the size and location of the hemorrhage. They may include dizziness, nausea, seizures, decreased sensations, hemiplegia, hemiparesis, aphasia, dysphagia, dysarthria, abnormal pupil size and response, visual field deficits, homonymous hemianopia, blindness, urinary incontinence, irregular respirations, positive Babinski's reflex, and decorticate or decerebrate posture. The patient's history may include cerebral aneurysm, congenital vascular defects, hemorrhagic disorders, head trauma, blood dyscrasias, or use of anticoagulants.

Meningitis. A patient who has this infection will experience a severe, constant, generalized headache that starts suddenly and worsens with movement. He may also have nuchal rigidity and a fever. Associated signs and symptoms include chills, positive Kernig's and Brudzinski's signs, hyperreflexia, and opisthotonos. As ICP increases, vomiting and occasionally papilledema develop. You may also detect an

altered LOC, seizures, ocular palsies, facial weakness, and hearing loss. The patient's history may include a previous systemic or sinus infection, dental work, or exposure to bacteria or viruses that commonly cause meningitis, such as *Haemophilus influenzae, Streptococcus pneumoniae, Neisseria meningitidis,* enteroviruses, and mumps virus.

Subarachnoid hemorrhage. The hallmarks of this disorder are a sudden, violent headache along with nuchal rigidity, dizziness, nausea, vomiting, seizures, hypertension, ipsilateral pupil dilation, and an altered LOC that may rapidly progress to coma. The patient may also have positive Kernig's and Brudzinski's signs, photophobia, blurred vision, and fever. Focal signs and symptoms, such as hemiparesis, hemiplegia, sensory or vision disturbances, and aphasia, may occur, as well as signs and symptoms of increased ICP. The patient's history may include congenital vascular defects, arteriovenous malformation, cardiovascular disease, smoking, or excessive stress.

Subdural hematoma. A severe, localized headache usually follows head trauma that causes an immediate loss of consciousness, a latent period of drowsiness, confusion or personality changes, and agitation. Later, indications of ICP may develop. Ipsilateral pupillary dilation progressing to fixation, coma, and focal neurologic deficits (such as hemiparesis) may also occur. If the patient's history includes head trauma within 3 days of the onset of symptoms, the hematoma is acute; within 3 weeks, subacute; and over 3 weeks, chronic. About 50% of patients with this disorder have no history of head trauma.

Other causes

Headache also results from certain causes that may not require immediate intervention.

Diagnostic tests. Pneumoencephalography may produce a severe generalized headache. Lumbar puncture or myelography may cause a throbbing frontal headache.

Disorders. A large number of headaches are migraine and cluster headaches, which recur periodically. A headache may also result from many common and some not-so-common conditions and disorders, including anxiety, eyestrain, acute sinusitis, influenza, fever, dehydration, hypertension, temporal arteritis, psittacosis, typhoid fever, and brain tumor. Headache may follow a concussion or seizure, and some persons get headaches simply from coughing, sneezing, heavy lifting, or stooping.

Drugs. A wide variety of drugs may cause headaches. These include nonsteroidal anti-inflammatory drugs, which cause morning headache in about half of all patients taking them; vasodilators (including nitrates and hydralazine), which typically cause a throbbing headache; cerebral stimulants such as amphetamine; skeletal muscle relaxants such as methocarbamol; antiemetics such as dimenhydrinate; anticholinergics such as propantheline; androgens; oral contraceptives; estrogens; progestogens; and some antihypertensives such as diazoxide. Headache may also follow the patient's withdrawal from ergot alkaloids, vasopressors, or sympathomimetic drugs like epinephrine. Ingestion of alcohol, particularly red wines, may cause headaches in some people.

Treatments. Cervical traction with pins commonly causes headache, which may be generalized or localized at the pin insertion sites.

Hematemesis

Hematemesis, or vomiting of blood, usually indicates bleeding in the GI tract above the ligament of Treitz, which suspends the duodenum at its junction with the jejunum. Bright red or blood-streaked vomitus signifies fresh or recent bleeding. Dark red, brown, or black vomitus — about the color and consistency of coffee grounds — indicates that blood has been retained in the stomach and partially digested.

Hematesis always indicates a serious problem — just how serious depends on the amount and source of the bleeding. Massive hematemesis (vomiting of 500 to 1,000 ml of blood) may indicate an immediate life-threatening situation. (See *Managing severe hematemesis,* pages 84 and 85, and *Selecting a tube for hematemesis control,* page 87.)

History questions

Explore the patient's problem by asking appropriate questions from this section. If the patient requires emergency intervention, continue collecting the history as you intervene or when he's stable.

• Have the patient describe the amount, color, and consistency of the vomitus. Find out how long he's been vomiting and if he's had a similar episode before. If so, when? How long did it last?

• Ask the patient if he's had any bloody or black, tarry stools with the hematemesis. Ask too about

EMERGENCY INTERVENTION

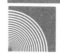

Managing severe hematemesis

Severe hematemesis may indicate acute intestinal bleeding—a medical emergency. If your patient loses more than 30% of his blood volume, hypovolemic shock will develop. But with accurate assessment and quick intervention, you can help prevent shock.

To determine how much blood the patient has lost, monitor his vital signs. If he's lost less than 15%, his vital signs probably won't change. Depending on his size, a loss of 1 liter of blood will usually trigger signs and symptoms of impending shock. So watch for tachycardia, a decrease in blood pressure, and orthostatic hypotension.

Use the tilt test to evaluate volume depletion. Have the patient rise from the prone position. As he does, check his pulse rate and blood pressure. If his pulse rate rises 10 beats/minute and his systolic blood pressure drops

10 mm Hg, then he's volume depleted. If he's in shock, you may need a Doppler flowmeter to check his blood pressure.

The best sign of poor perfusion is delayed capillary refill time (greater than 2 seconds). A rapid, thready pulse; cool and clammy skin; restlessness; confusion; and worsening hypotension indicate hypovolemic shock.

If the patient shows signs of impending shock (or if he's already in shock), your first priority is to ensure perfusion of his vital organs—particularly the heart and brain. Place him flat and insert a large-bore I.V. line for emergency fluid and blood replacement. Initially, you'll give normal saline solution or lactated Ringer's solution. For impending shock, add a colloidal volume expander, such as Plasmanate, if the blood transfusion will be delayed. But a transfusion of whole

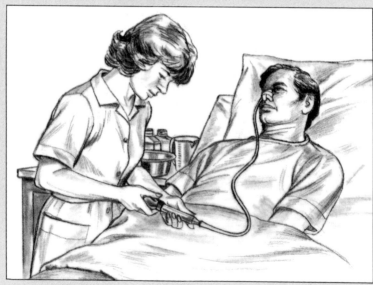

Using a nasogastric tube to aspirate stomach contents

blood or packed red blood cells is the only way to replace the blood's oxygen-carrying capacity.

Prepare to have blood samples drawn for hemoglobin, hematocrit, blood urea nitrogen, electrolyte, and prothrombin time tests as well as for blood typing and cross matching. Begin oxygen therapy to ensure maximum oxygen saturation of available hemoglobin, and monitor oxygen saturation using pulse oximetry. Insert an indwelling urinary catheter to monitor urine output. Also, insert a nasogastric tube (such as the Sengstaken-Blakemore, Ewald, or Salem sump). This will be used to aspirate stomach contents, evaluate the bleeding, and possibly lavage the stomach until the contents are clear (see illustration).

Continue monitoring the patient for signs of shock, changes in his level of consciousness, angina, ECG changes indicating inadequate myocardial oxygenation, and low urine output indicating hypovolemia or impaired renal function. The patient's hourly urine output should be at least 0.5 ml/kg or about 30 ml. Central venous pressure or pulmonary capillary wedge pressure reflects fluid volume status more accurately than urine output. So the doctor may want to insert a central venous or pulmonary artery catheter.

Remember that individual assessment findings, such as a low blood pressure reading, aren't necessarily significant. Rather, it's the *change* in one or more findings that can indicate a significant shift in the patient's condition.

Prepare the patient for probable endoscopy. Explain what to expect during the procedure and how it will help the doctor find the source of the bleeding. Once the doctor makes a diagnosis, treatment of the underlying cause can begin.

associated pain and have him describe its location and quality.
• Has the patient had other associated symptoms — such as nausea, flatulence, diarrhea, weakness, malaise, dyspnea, palpitations, faintness, thirst, sweating, syncope, or difficulty eating or swallowing — before or since the onset of vomiting?
• When did the patient last eat? How much did he eat? Has he ingested any caustic substances? If so, he may have been attempting suicide.
• Ask how much alcohol the patient drinks, on average, in a day or a week. Find out if he's experiencing any unusual stress. Has he recently had severe trauma, illness, burns, central nervous system trauma or surgery, or sepsis?
• Does he have a history of epigastric distress? If so, is it usually relieved by food or antacids? Determine whether he has a history of peptic ulcers, or liver or coagulation disorders. If he has one of these problems, does he comply with his medical regimen?
• Is he currently taking aspirin or other nonsteroidal anti-inflammatory drugs (such as phenylbutazone or indomethacin), corticosteroids, or drugs that impair coagulation?

Physical examination

Base your assessment of the patient on the health history information you've collected. Assess his abdomen, making sure you auscultate before palpating and percussing. Using this alternative sequence ensures that you don't affect the frequency or intensity of bowel sounds before you assess them.

Inspection. Look carefully at the patient's skin, noting its color, temperature, and any sweating, turgor, or signs of bleeding or burns. Examine the mucous membranes of the mouth and nasopharynx, again looking for turgor, bleeding, or burns. Then check for neck edema. Observe the rate and depth of the patient's breathing. Is he having difficulty breathing? Is he exhibiting an abnormal breathing pattern?

Auscultation. Listen for bowel sounds, noting any abnormalities. Next, auscultate the lungs for adventitious sounds, such as crackles, rhonchi, or diminished breath sounds. As you monitor the patient's blood pressure and pulse pressure, note any changes.

Palpation. Gently palpate the abdomen for tenderness and pain. Then palpate the neck and anterior chest for subcutaneous crepitus. Check too for lymphadenopathy. As you palpate the peripheral pulses, note their rate, rhythm, and intensity.

Percussion. Lightly percuss the abdomen for rebound tenderness or pain.

Life-threatening causes
Your assessment may lead you to suspect one or more of the following.

Erosive gastritis. Coffee-ground or bright red hematemesis may be the only symptom of this disorder. Or the patient may also have abdominal pain, nausea, and vomiting. His history may include chronic ingestion of aspirin, nonsteroidal anti-inflammatory drugs, corticosteroids, or alcohol, or ingestion of caustic agents — possibly used in a suicide attempt.

Esophageal injury by caustics. Ingestion of a caustic agent inevita-

bly produces some esophageal damage. The grossly bloody or coffee-ground hematemesis is accompanied by prostration and severe mouth, epigastric, and anterior or retrosternal chest pain that's intensified by swallowing. You may see burns on the patient's oropharynx. If he hasn't sought help for 3 or 4 weeks, dysphagia, marked salivation, and fever may have developed. These symptoms worsen as esophageal strictures form. The patient's history will reveal recent ingestion of corrosive acid or alkali.

Esophageal or gastric varices (ruptured). With this disorder, hematemesis may be massive and bright red or have a coffee-ground appearance. The patient may show signs of shock, such as hypotension and tachycardia, after hematemesis — or even before, if his stomach filled with blood before he vomited. He may also report melena or painless hematochezia, ranging from slight oozing to massive rectal hemorrhage. The patient's history may reveal chronic alcoholism, portal hypertension, or esophageal varices. In a patient with esophageal varices, nasogastric intubation may cause their rupture.

Esophageal rupture from Boerhaave's syndrome. Most common in men, this rupture is characterized by severe hematemesis accompanied by excessive vomiting, coughing, or retching. The patient also has severe retrosternal, epigastric, neck, or scapular pain and edema of the chest and neck. He may show signs of respiratory distress. Your examination will reveal subcutaneous emphysema in the chest wall, supraclavicular fossa, and neck. The patient may have eaten a large meal recently.

Selecting a tube for hematemesis control

When your patient has hematemesis, you'll need to help insert a nasogastric tube. This procedure allows blood drainage, aspiration of stomach contents, or gastric lavage. Knowing the advantages of each of the commonly used tubes will help you anticipate the most appropriate one for your patient's needs.

Small-bore gastric tubes

The Salem sump tube (shown at right), a double-lumen nasogastric tube, is used to remove stomach contents and perform gastric lavage. Because of its small bore, this tube may be inadequate if you're trying to lavage large amounts of fluid rapidly. The small bore also prohibits aspiration of large blood clots. The main advantage of the small bore is the patient's comfort.

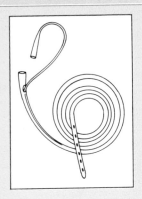

The double-lumen is preferable to a single-lumen tube because it allows atmospheric air to enter the patient's stomach. Thus, the tube can float freely, reducing the risk of adhesions and damage to the gastric mucosa.

Wide-bore gastric tubes

The Ewald tube has a wide bore that allows clots and large amounts of fluid to pass quickly. It's especially useful with patients who have massive GI bleeding. Another wide-bore tube, the double-lumen Levacutor, has a large lumen for evacuation of gastric contents and a small one for lavage. The Edlich tube (shown at right) has one wide-bore lumen with four openings near the closed distal tip. A funnel or syringe can be connected at the proximal end. Like the other tubes, the Edlich can aspirate a large volume rapidly.

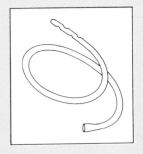

Esophageal tubes

The Sengstaken-Blakemore tube (shown at right) is a triple-lumen, double-balloon esophageal tube. It has a gastric aspiration port that allows for contents to drain below the gastric balloon. The gastric balloon can be inflated to compress bleeding vessels and help stop the bleeding. A similar tube, the Linton, lacks an esophageal balloon. With it, you can aspirate esophageal and gastric contents without risking necrosis. The Minnesota esophagogastric tamponade tube, which has four lumens and two balloons, provides pressure monitoring ports for both balloons without the need for Y connectors.

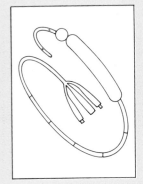

Esophagitis. With this disorder, the patient's hematemesis may be bright red or have a coffee-ground appearance. Usually, the hematemesis is accompanied by odynophagia and dysphagia. The patient's history may include chronic alcoholism or irradiation of the esophagus.

Mallory-Weiss syndrome. In this disorder, coffee-ground or bright-vomiting, retching, or straining (as from coughing). The severe bleeding may cause hypovolemic shock, and you may note tachycardia, hypotension, dyspnea, and cool, clammy skin. The patient's history may include excessive alcohol ingestion.

Peptic ulcers. An ulcer penetrating into an artery can result in massive hematemesis of bright red blood. Other symptoms include melena or hematochezia, chills, fever, and signs of shock and dehydration (such as tachycardia, hypotension, poor skin turgor, and thirst). The patient's history may or may not reveal peptic ulcer disease. He may report only gastric pain that's relieved by foods or antacids, nausea, vomiting, and epigastric tenderness. If the patient knows he has peptic ulcer disease, he may not be complying with his medical regimen. His history may include alcoholism; a recent episode of excessive stress from severe trauma, illness, or burns; central nervous system trauma or surgery; or sepsis.

Other causes
Certain causes of hematemesis may not require immediate intervention.

Disorders. Hematemesis can occur with gastric polyps, benign and malignant tumors, vascular malfor-

mations, hemobilia, inflammatory bowel disease, diverticula, Peutz-Jeghers syndrome, Osler-Weber-Rendu disease, and hemorrhagic disease of the newborn.

Drugs. Chronic use of aspirin, non-steroidal anti-inflammatory drugs, and ethacrynic acid as well as large doses of reserpine may cause gastric hemorrhage. Anticoagulant medication can produce bleeding diathesis.

Treatments. Hematemesis may follow oropharyngeal or nasal surgery if the patient has swallowed blood.

Hemoptysis

Expectoration of blood or bloody sputum from the lungs or tracheobronchial tree is known as hemoptysis. Usually resulting from abnormalities of the tracheobronchial tree, hemoptysis is associated with inflammatory conditions or lesions that cause erosion and necrosis of the bronchial tissues and blood vessels. Hemoptysis can also be caused by diapedesis of red blood cells from the pulmonary microvasculature into the alveoli. Sometimes, hemoptysis can be confused with bleeding from the mouth, throat, nasopharynx, or GI tract (see *Identifying hemoptysis*).

If your patient is expectorating large amounts of blood, anticipate helping with emergency endotracheal intubation and suctioning (see *Controlling massive hemoptysis*, page 90).

History questions
Explore the patient's problem by asking appropriate questions from

this section. If the patient requires emergency intervention, continue collecting the history as you intervene or when he's stable.

• Try to determine how much blood the patient is coughing up and how often. Ask when the hemoptysis began and if the patient has ever had a similar episode before.

• Does he have any associated symptoms, such as nausea, vomiting, fever, dyspnea, dysphagia, hoarseness, a productive or nonproductive cough, or pain in the chest, neck, or abdomen? If he reports associated pain, have him describe it and indicate its location.

• Find out if he has recently had a flulike syndrome with such symptoms as headache, anorexia, fever and chills, weakness, and weight loss. What about any recent invasive pulmonary procedures—such as bronchoscopy, laryngoscopy, or lung biopsy?

• Ask the patient if he smokes or if he ever smoked. How many packs a day does he (or did he) smoke? For how long?

• Determine if he has a history of chest trauma, varicose veins, thrombophlebitis, or cardiac, pulmonary, or bleeding disorders. Has he recently had pneumonia or hip or leg fractures? How about prolonged bed rest?

• What medications is the patient taking? Particularly note any drugs that can increase the risk of bleeding, such as aspirin and anticoagulants. If the patient is a woman, ask if she's using oral contraceptives.

Physical examination
Base your assessment of the patient on the health history information you've collected.

Inspection. Examine the patient's nose, mouth, and pharynx for

Identifying hemoptysis

These guidelines will help you distinguish hemoptysis from epistaxis, hematemesis, and brown, red, or pink sputum.

Hemoptysis

Often frothy because it's mixed with air, the expectorated fluid will usually be bright red. If you test it with litmus paper, you'll find it has an alkaline pH.

Associated respiratory signs and symptoms strongly suggest hemoptysis. These include a cough, a tickling sensation in the throat, and blood produced by repeated coughing.

You can rule out epistaxis because the patient's nasal passages and posterior pharynx are usually clear.

Hematemesis

Hematemesis originates in the GI tract. The patient vomits or regurgitates either bright red blood or material that has a coffee-ground appearance because it has been retained in the stomach and partially digested. The vomitus may contain food particles. It'll test positive for occult blood, and you'll find it has an acidic pH. After an episode of hematemesis, the patient's stool may show traces of blood. Many patients with hematemesis complain of dyspepsia.

Brown, red, or pink sputum

Oxidation of inhaled bronchodilators can produce brown, red, or pink sputum. Sputum that resembles old blood may come from rupture of an ameba-caused abscess into the bronchus. Red or brown sputum may also be seen when a patient has pneumonia caused by the enterobacterium *Serratia marcescens*.

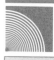

Controlling massive hemoptysis

Massive hemoptysis can cause airway obstruction, asphyxiation, and hypovolemic shock.

Your first priority is to monitor vital signs for impending shock. Check for an increase of 10 beats/minute in pulse rate and a decrease of 10 mm Hg in systolic blood pressure when the patient rises from a prone to a sitting position.

Next, insert a large-bore I.V. line for fluid replacement and administration of emergency drugs and blood components, which will be ordered to prevent or treat shock. Give oxygen to ensure that the patient gets the maximum oxygenation from his available hemoglobin.

Obtain arterial blood samples for arterial blood gas analysis and venous blood samples for hemoglobin, hematocrit, blood urea nitrogen, electrolyte, and prothrombin time tests, as well as for blood typing and cross matching.

Be ready to help with emergency bronchoscopy, which will be performed to identify the bleeding site and clear the airway.

cyanosis or pallor. Test whether capillary refill is delayed more than 2 seconds. Also, assess the patient's level of consciousness, looking for such signs and symptoms as restlessness, anxiety, lethargy, stupor, or coma.

Palpation. Check the rate, rhythm, and intensity of the peripheral pulses. As you palpate the patient's chest, note the level of the diaphragm and any tenderness, respiratory excursion, fremitus, or abnormal pulsations. If the patient has a history of trauma, carefully check the position of the trachea and note any edema.

Percussion. Check the lungs for flatness, dullness, hyperresonance, or tympany.

Auscultation. In all lung fields, note the quality and intensity of breath sounds and listen for crackles, rhonchi, and wheezes. Next, auscultate the heart for murmurs, gallops, bruits, and pleural friction rubs. Monitor the patient's blood pressure and pulse pressure.

Life-threatening causes
Your assessment may lead you to suspect one or more of the following.

Aortic aneurysm (ruptured). When this rupture occurs, hemoptysis is sudden, massive, and projectile. Death is imminent. The patient may have signs and symptoms of a dissecting aortic aneurysm before hemoptysis begins. These would include the sudden onset of extremely severe chest and neck pain, radiating to the upper back, abdomen, and lower back. The chest pain is often described as excruciating, tearing, ripping, or stabbing. If the

sources of bleeding. For instance, check for poor oral or dental hygiene or gingivitis. Note the color, consistency, and odor of all expectorated sputum.

Now, observe the rate and depth of the patient's respirations. Is he having difficulty breathing? Do you note any changes from the normal respiratory pattern? Observe his chest configuration. As he breathes, look for abnormal movement, accessory muscle use, and retractions. Note whether his neck veins are distended.

Inspect the skin for lesions, diaphoresis, and central or peripheral patient reports dull pain (or no pain), compromised neurologic function may be decreasing his perception of the pain or his ability to complain about it. His history may include cardiovascular disease or chest pain.

Lung abscess. A patient with this lesion will expectorate copious amounts of bloody, purulent, and foul-smelling sputum. He's also likely to have fever with chills, diaphoresis, anorexia, weight loss, headache, weakness, dyspnea, and pleuritic or dull chest pain. When you auscultate his chest, you'll find tubular or cavernous breath sounds and crackles. Percussion reveals dullness on the affected side. The patient's history may include recent pulmonary infection or evidence of poor oral hygiene with dental or gingival disease.

Pulmonary edema. With this disorder, a dyspneic patient may expectorate copious amounts of pink, frothy sputum. This may be preceded by signs of congestive heart failure, such as distended neck veins and orthopnea. Other signs and symptoms include tachycardia, tachypnea, S_3 gallop, crackles in both lung fields, thready pulse, oliguria, hypotension, diaphoresis, cyanosis, productive or nonproductive cough, and marked anxiety. The patient's history may include cardiovascular disease or dyspneic episodes with an abrupt or gradual onset, fatigue, weight gain, pallor or cyanosis, diaphoresis, and anxiety.

Pulmonary embolism with infarction. Blood-tinged sputum and, less commonly, massive hemoptysis may occur with the sudden dyspnea that's the hallmark of this disorder. Also characteristic is intense angina

or pleuritic chest pain aggravated by deep breathing and thoracic movement. If the embolus is large enough to cause significant obstruction of the pulmonary circulation, central cyanosis occurs. You may also note anxiety, tachycardia, tachypnea, productive or nonproductive cough, low-grade fever, restlessness, diaphoresis, crackles, pleural friction rub, diffuse wheezing, dull percussion sounds, signs of circulatory collapse (weak, rapid pulse and hypotension), signs of cerebral ischemia (transient unconsciousness, coma, seizures), signs of hypoxia (restlessness), and—particularly if the patient is elderly—hemiplegia and other focal neurologic deficits. Less commonly, you'll detect such signs and symptoms as chest splinting, leg edema, and distended neck veins. The patient's history may include any of the following: thrombophlebitis of the deep systemic veins, varicose veins, hip or leg fractures, acute myocardial infarction, congestive heart failure, cardiogenic shock, congestive cardiomyopathies, pregnancy, or use of oral contraceptives.

Tracheal trauma. The bleeding will appear to come from the back of the throat with this disorder. Accompanying signs and symptoms may include hoarseness, dysphagia, neck pain, airway occlusion, and respiratory distress. The patient will have experienced anterior neck trauma.

Other causes
Certain causes of hemoptysis may not require immediate intervention.

Diagnostic tests. Bronchoscopy, laryngoscopy, mediastinoscopy, or lung biopsy can cause lung or airway injury that produces hemoptysis.

Disorders. Hemoptysis can occur if the patient has bronchiectasis, bronchitis, lung carcinoma, cystic fibrosis, Goodpasture's syndrome, idiopathic pulmonary hemosiderosis, pulmonary contusion, pulmonary cysts, or tuberculosis.

Hyperpnea

When a person increases his respiratory effort for a sustained period, he has hyperpnea. He may be breathing at a normal rate (at least 12 breaths/minute) but with increased depth (a tidal volume greater than 500 ml). Or he may be breathing at an increased rate (more than 20 breaths/minute) but with normal depth. Or both the rate and depth of his breathing may be increased.

Hyperpnea differs from sighing, a term that refers to intermittent deep inspirations. Hyperpnea can, however, be called tachypnea when the depth of a patient's respirations remains normal but his respiratory rate increases.

Typically, a patient with hyperpnea breathes at a normal or an increased rate and inhales deeply, displaying marked chest expansion. The patient may complain of shortness of breath if the problem stems from a respiratory disorder causing hypoxemia. If, however, the patient's problem results from either a metabolic or neurologic disorder, he may not be aware of his abnormal breathing.

Hyperpnea that results from a severe head injury is called central neurogenic hyperventilation. Whether its onset is acute or gradual, this type of hyperpnea indicates damage to the lower midbrain or upper pons. You'll note that both the rate and depth of respirations increase.

Acute intermittent hyperventilation may be a response to hypoxemia, anxiety, fear, pain, or excitement. An excessive inhalation of carbon dioxide may cause hyperpnea associated with respiratory alkalosis. Another form of hyperpnea, Kussmaul's respirations occur as a compensatory response to excessive carbon dioxide levels (see *Kussmaul's respirations: A compensatory mechanism*).

History questions
Explore the patient's problem by asking appropriate questions from this section.
• Did the hyperpnea start suddenly or gradually? Was it preceded by a specific event? For example, did the patient consume a lot of alcohol or ethylene glycol?
• Find out if the patient has any associated symptoms—headache, fatigue, changes in his level of consciousness, nausea, seizures, syncope, or paresthesia.
• Determine if he's recently had a disorder that caused a loss of bicarbonate, such as severe diarrhea or vomiting, or if he's recently undergone GI suctioning.
• Does the patient have a history of dieting, anorexia nervosa, bulimia, or starvation? When did he last eat?
• Does the patient have a history of disorders that could predispose him to metabolic acidosis—for instance, diabetes mellitus or renal disease? What about any underlying cardiac, pulmonary, or thyroid disorders?
• Ask if the patient is taking any medications—especially paraldehyde, carbonic anhydrase inhibitors, anion-exchange resins, or salicylates.

Kussmaul's respirations: A compensatory mechanism

The term *Kussmaul's respirations* describes fast, deep breathing without pauses that characteristically sounds labored. The deep breaths resemble sighs. This breathing pattern develops when respiratory centers in the medulla detect decreased blood pH. That triggers the compensatory fast, deep breathing to remove excess carbon dioxide and restore the pH balance.

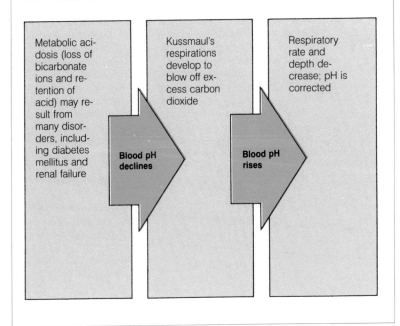

Metabolic acidosis (loss of bicarbonate ions and retention of acid) may result from many disorders, including diabetes mellitus and renal failure

Blood pH declines

Kussmaul's respirations develop to blow off excess carbon dioxide

Blood pH rises

Respiratory rate and depth decrease; pH is corrected

Physical examination

Base your assessment of the patient on the health history information you've collected.

Inspection. Note the rate and depth of the patient's breathing. Is the respiratory pattern abnormal? Check for intercostal and abdominal retractions, use of accessory muscles, and diaphoresis.

Next, observe for cyanosis, especially of the mouth, lips, mucous membranes, and earlobes, and for alterations in the level of consciousness (restlessness, anxiety, lethargy, and stupor) — all signs of decreased tissue oxygenation. While checking the patient's skin and mucous membranes, note any turgor, which may indicate dehydration. Inspect his head and face for signs of trauma.

Does the patient have an abnormal pupillary response, indicating increased intracranial pressure (ICP)? Inspect his abdomen for ascites, draining wounds, and signs of infection.

Palpation. If you suspect a head injury, gently palpate the patient's

What causes metabolic acidosis and respiratory alkalosis

Metabolic acidosis and respiratory alkalosis can result from many causes.

Metabolic acidosis

Metabolic acidosis can stem from any condition that makes pH acidic. These conditions include:
- diabetic ketoacidosis
- ethylene glycol
- ethanol, methanol, paraldehyde, or salicylate intoxication
- high-fat diets
- renal failure
- sepsis
- shock
- starvation
- tissue hypoxia.

Metabolic acidosis can also stem from bicarbonate loss, caused by:
- anion-exchange resins, carbonic anhydrase inhibitors, or chloride-containing acids, such as hydrochloric acid
- draining fistulas of the pancreas or small bowel
- extracellular fluid-volume expansion
- GI suctioning or profuse dehydration, diarrhea, or vomiting
- hyperalimentation
- ileal conduit or ureterosigmoidostomy
- renal tubular acidosis

Respiratory alkalosis

Respiratory alkalosis may stem from any of these conditions:
- alcohol, paraldehyde, or salicylate intoxication
- anemia
- anxiety
- brain lesions
- cirrhosis
- congestive heart failure
- encephalitis
- exercise
- fever

- head trauma
- hypoxia
- hysteria
- mechanical hyperventilation
- meningitis
- pulmonary fibrosis
- sepsis caused by gram-negative organisms
- thyrotoxicosis
- voluntary hyperpnea (to relieve pain or stress).

head for fractures. As you palpate his peripheral pulses, note their rate, rhythm, and intensity.

Percussion. Next, percuss for carpopedal spasm.

Auscultation. Listen for adventitious breath sounds and for an irregular heart rhythm. Then monitor the patient's blood pressure and pulse pressure.

Life-threatening causes
Your assessment may lead you to

suspect one or more of the following.

Head injury. A sudden or gradual onset of hyperpnea will be accompanied by signs and symptoms reflecting the site and extent of the injury. These may include loss of consciousness; soft-tissue injury; bony deformity of the face, head, or neck; facial edema; clear or bloody drainage from the mouth, nose, or ears; raccoon's eyes; Battle's sign; an absent doll's eye sign; and motor and sensory disturbances. Signs of increased ICP include a decreased response to painful stimuli, loss of pupillary reaction, bradycardia, increased systolic pressure, and widening pulse pressure. The patient's history reveals head trauma.

Metabolic acidosis. This condition is characterized by Kussmaul's respirations, which can occur abruptly or gradually, depending on the underlying disorder. The abnormal breathing may be accompanied by drowsiness, decreased mental function (including confusion, coma, and seizures), hypotension, tissue hypoxia, cardiac dysrhythmias, anorexia, nausea, and vomiting. You may also note fruity breath if the patient is diabetic or alcohol breath if he has consumed a large amount of alcohol. The patient's history will include conditions that lead to loss of bicarbonate ions or disorders that produce excessive levels of acid in the body (see *What causes metabolic acidosis and respiratory alkalosis*).

Respiratory alkalosis. The patient will experience hyperventilation, which may be episodic. His arterial pH will be above 7.45 and his partial pressure of carbon dioxide in arterial blood below 35 mm Hg. The patient may also experience breathlessness, vertigo, syncope, nervousness, paresthesias of the extremities, perioral paresthesia, muscle cramps and tetany, seizures, decreased mentation, confusion, decreased psychomotor performance, anxiety, cardiac dysrhythmias, and hypotension. The patient's history will include a disorder that decreases carbon dioxide levels in the blood.

Other causes
Hyperpnea may also accompany strenuous exercise. A person who's experiencing stress or pain or a woman who's in labor may use voluntary hyperpnea to relax.

Hypertension

An intermittent or sustained increase in blood pressure exceeding 140/86 mm Hg constitutes hypertension, commonly called high blood pressure. The condition may develop suddenly or gradually.

A sudden rise in blood pressure to 200/120 mm Hg indicates a life-threatening hypertensive crisis (see *Managing elevated blood pressure,* page 96). A less dramatic increase, which may have developed over a span of years, may be cause for concern but isn't necessarily an emergency. (For information on the pathophysiology of hypertension, see *Understanding elevated blood pressure,* pages 98 and 99.)

History questions
Explore the patient's problem by asking appropriate questions from this section. If the patient requires emergency intervention, continue collecting the history as you intervene or when he's stable.
• Does the patient have any symptoms? Ask specifically about headaches — particularly suboccipital headaches when he wakes up in the morning. Also, ask if he's experiencing palpitations, sweating, nausea, vomiting, epistaxis, urinary burning, or decreased urine output. If he has symptoms, what was he doing when they began?
• Has he had similar episodes? If so, was the precipitating event the same? Did anything help relieve the symptoms or the rise in blood pressure?

Managing elevated blood pressure

Elevated blood pressure can signal various life-threatening disorders. If blood pressure exceeds 200/120 mm Hg, the patient is experiencing a hypertensive crisis and needs immediate treatment.

First, have another nurse notify the doctor at once. Maintain a patent airway in case the patient vomits. Begin seizure precautions, and prepare to administer antihypertensive drugs and diuretics I.V. Also, insert an indwelling urinary (Foley) catheter to accurately monitor urine output.

If blood pressure is less severely elevated, continue to rule out other life-threatening causes. If your patient is pregnant, suspect preeclampsia or eclampsia. Have her rest in bed. Insert an I.V line and be ready to administer magnesium sulfate, which decreases neuromuscular irritability, and antihypertensives, as ordered. Monitor the patient's vital signs closely for the next 24 hours. If her diastolic blood pressure stays above 100 mm Hg despite drug therapy, the doctor may induce labor or perform a cesarean section. During this time, provide emotional support.

If your patient isn't pregnant, look for other clues to the cause of hypertension. Observe for exophthalmos and an enlarged thyroid gland. If you find them, ask the patient about a history of hyperthyroidism. Then check for other associated signs and symptoms, including tachycardia, widened pulse pressure, palpitations, severe weakness, diarrhea, a temperature above 100° F (37.8° C), and nervousness. Report these findings immediately to the doctor. Prepare to administer antithyroid drugs orally or by nasogastric tube, if necessary. Also, evaluate the patient's fluid status, looking for signs of dehydration, such as poor skin turgor. If you find such signs, the patient may require I.V. fluid replacement and temperature control with a hypothermia blanket.

If your patient shows signs of increased intracranial pressure (such as a decreased level of consciousness and fixed or dilated pupils), ask if he's experienced head trauma recently. Then check for increased respirations and bradycardia. Report these signs immediately to the doctor. Maintain a patent airway in case the patient vomits. Institute seizure precautions, and prepare to give diuretics I.V. Insert a Foley catheter, and monitor fluid intake and output. Check the patient's vital signs every 15 minutes until they're stable.

If your patient's peripheral pulses are absent or weak, ask if he has chest pressure or pain, which would suggest a dissecting aortic aneurysm. Encourage bed rest until the doctor establishes a diagnosis. You may have to give the patient antihypertensives I.V., as ordered, or prepare him for surgery.

• If the patient is pregnant, find out if she has experienced a sudden weight gain and generalized edema over the last month. Note the gestational age of the fetus.
• Has the patient recently experienced unusual stress — perhaps from an infection, surgery, or physical or emotional trauma? Does he smoke? If so, how much? How long has he been smoking? Is he on a special diet? How well does he tolerate heat?
• Determine if the patient has a history or a family history of hypertension. Does he have a history of

renal, cardiac, or endocrine disease? What about claudication?

• Is the patient taking a medication that could elevate his blood pressure? These medications include albuterol, epinephrine, isocarboxazid, amphetamines, sympathomimetic drugs, corticosteroids, and over-the-counter nasal decongestants. If the patient is taking a monoamine oxidase inhibitor, find out if he has ingested any substance containing tyramine, such as aged cheese, yeast, beer, or wine. If the patient is a woman, ask if she's taking oral contraceptives.

Physical examination

Base your assessment of the patient on the health history information you've collected.

Inspection. Note the rate and depth of the patient's breathing and any changes from normal respiratory patterns. As he breathes, look for excursion.

Inspect skin color and temperature. Then check for decreased skin turgor and diaphoresis. To determine the patient's hydration status, inspect his mucous membranes. Check his arms and legs for edema and adequate capillary refill time. Does he have exophthalmos or jugular vein distention?

Examine a urine sample for turbidity or hematuria and any expectorations for pink, frothy sputum. Note any neuromuscular irritability, such as spasms or fasciculations.

Palpation. Check the rate, rhythm, intensity, and characteristics of the peripheral pulses. As you palpate the aortic area, note any pulsating mass. If you don't suspect pheochromocytoma as the cause of hypertension, palpate the abdomen for rigidity, tenderness, and hepato-

megaly. Check the flank area and costovertebral angle for edema, tenderness, and kidney enlargement. Feel the thyroid to determine its position and size.

Percussion. Next, percuss the abdomen to detect liver enlargement.

Auscultation. To establish that the patient's blood pressure is actually elevated, you may need serial readings or readings taken with the patient both supine and standing. Continue monitoring the patient's blood pressure and pulse pressure. Be sure to compare each reading with your baseline measurement.

Auscultate for any diminished or abnormal heart sounds—gallops, murmurs, or ejection clicks, for example. Listen over the lung fields to detect any abnormal breath sounds, such as crackles or wheezes. As you auscultate over the carotid artery, abdomen, flank, and costovertebral angle, note any bruits. Check each abdominal quadrant for bowel sounds.

Life-threatening causes

Your assessment may lead you to suspect one or more of the following.

Aortic aneurysm (dissecting). Initially, the patient will have a sudden rise in systolic pressure but no change in diastolic pressure. The increase is short-lived, however; the body's ability to compensate fails, resulting in hypotension. Associated signs amd symptoms depend on whether the aneurysm is in the abdomen or thorax.

With an abdominal aneurysm, the patient may have persistent abdominal and back pain, weakness, sweating, tachycardia, dyspnea, restlessness, confusion, cool and

Understanding elevated blood pressure

Blood pressure—the force blood exerts on vessels as it flows through them—depends on cardiac output, peripheral resistance, and blood volume. A brief review of the regulating mechanisms will help you understand how elevated blood pressure develops. These mechanisms are nervous system control, capillary fluid shifts, kidney excretion, and hormonal changes.

Elevated blood pressure signals the breakdown or inappropriate response of these pressure-regulating mechanisms. Its associated signs and symptoms are reflected in the target organs and tissues illustrated.

Nervous system control

The brain stem influences the sympathetic division, composed chiefly of baroreceptors (B) and chemoreceptors (C). These receptors promote moderate vasoconstriction to maintain normal blood pressure. When these receptors don't respond appropriately, increased vasoconstriction occurs, enhancing peripheral resistance and resulting in elevated blood pressure.

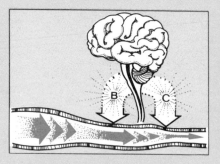

Capillary fluid shifts

These shifts regulate blood volume by responding to arterial pressure. Increased pressure forces fluid into the interstitial spaces; decreased pressure allows it to be drawn back into the arteries. However, this fluid shift may take several hours to adjust the blood pressure.

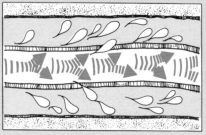

clammy skin, mottled skin below the waist, absent femoral and pedal pulses, increasing abdominal girth, and abdominal rigidity. Your auscultation may reveal a systolic bruit. When you palpate the abdomen, you may find tenderness over the area of the aneurysm and an epigastric mass that will be pulsating if it hasn't yet ruptured.

With a thoracic aneurysm, the patient may complain of severe ripping or tearing pain in the chest that may radiate to the neck, shoulders, lower back, or abdomen. Other signs and symptoms include pallor, syncope, sweating, dyspnea, tachycardia, cyanosis, leg weakness, and a sudden onset of neurologic symptoms. Your auscultation may reveal a murmur suggesting aortic regurgitation. In many cases, the patient's history will include smoking and claudication as well as other

Renal excretion

The kidneys help regulate blood volume by increasing or decreasing urine formation. Normally, a mean arterial pressure of about 60 mm Hg maintains urine output. When pressure drops below this level, urine formation ceases, thus increasing blood volume. Conversely, when arterial pressure exceeds 60 mm Hg, urine formation increases, thereby reducing blood volume. Like capillary fluid shifts, this mechanism may take several hours to adjust the blood pressure.

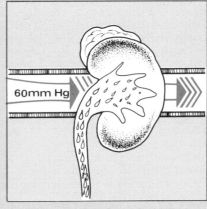

Hormonal changes

The kidneys' renin-angiotensin system responds to low arterial pressure by forming angiotensin (A_2). This hormone causes vasoconstriction, which increases arterial pressure. Angiotensin also stimulates the release of aldosterone (A), which regulates sodium retention—a key determinant of blood volume.

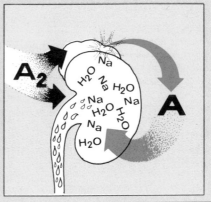

signs and symptoms of cardiovascular disease.

Hypertension (malignant). With this disorder, the patient will have an abrupt increase in diastolic pressure to above 120 mm Hg and in systolic pressure to above 200 mm Hg. This is characteristically accompanied by acute hypertensive retinopathy, malignant nephrosclerosis, or hypertensive encephalopathy. If the patient has cardiac disease, he'll also have pulmonary edema marked by neck vein distention, dyspnea, tachypnea, tachycardia, and a cough that produces pink, frothy sputum. Other signs and symptoms reflecting associated disorders may include a severe headache, confusion, coma, slurred speech, blurred vision, anxiety, retinal changes, tinnitus, epistaxis, muscle twitching, nausea, and vomiting. Your auscultation may reveal a diastolic murmur, a gallop, an irregular heart rhythm, bruits, or ejection clicks. You may hear crackles when you auscultate the lungs. On palpation, you may find the thyroid, liver, or kidneys enlarged, or you may note a mass over the abdominal aorta. The family history commonly includes malignant hypertension.

Increased intracranial pressure.
Initially, systolic blood pressure rises, and the patient experiences tachycardia, tachypnea or apneustic respirations, and a widening pulse pressure. Later, bradycardia and Cheyne-Stokes respirations or apnea develop. The patient may have such associated signs and symptoms as persistent headache, projectile vomiting, progressive loss of consciousness, seizures, and pupillary changes. The patient's history may reveal any of the following: head trauma, systemic infection, brain tumor, or underlying metabolic or cardiac disease.

Myocardial infarction. Blood pressure may either rise or fall when a myocardial infarction (MI) occurs. The disorder is characterized by crushing chest pain that may radiate to the jaw, shoulder, arm, or epigastrium. This pain may be accompanied by dyspnea, anxiety, nausea, vomiting, weakness, diaphoresis, and cyanotic or cool, pale skin. On auscultation, you may detect an atrial gallop or murmur and, occasionally, an irregular pulse rate. The patient may have a history or family history of cardiac disease. He may have recently experienced unusual stress or may have a lifestyle that includes excessive sodium and fat intake, lack of exercise, and smoking. He may also use cocaine, which can cause an MI.

Pheochromocytoma. A patient with this tumor can have a paroxysmal or sustained rise in blood pressure that may be accompanied by postural hypotension stemming from the release of catecholamines. Associated signs and symptoms may include anxiety, diaphoresis, palpitations, tremors, pallor, nausea, weight loss, and headache. A pregnant patient may report an increase in attacks as gestation progresses. That's because the enlarging uterus puts more and more pressure on the tumor. The patient's history may include episodes of hypertension, headache, sweating, and tachycardia.

Pregnancy-induced hypertension.
This disorder is defined as a blood pressure of 140/90 mm Hg or more during the first trimester of pregnancy, 130/80 mm Hg or more during the second or third trimester, or an increase of 30 mm Hg above the woman's baseline systolic pressure or 15 mm Hg above the baseline diastolic pressure at any time during the pregnancy. Along with the elevated blood pressure, the patient typically has generalized edema, a sudden weight gain of 3 lbs or more per week during the second or third trimester, severe frontal headache, blurred or double vision, decreased urine output or oliguria, midabdominal pain, neuromuscular irritability, nausea, and possibly seizures (eclampsia). The patient's history may reveal preeclampsia in previous pregnancies, hypertension, diabetes mellitus, or multiple parity.

Renovascular stenosis. Characteristic of this disorder is an abrupt rise in systolic and diastolic blood pressure along with bruits over the upper abdomen or the costovertebral angle, hematuria, and acute flank pain. Auscultation may reveal a high-pitched, systolic-diastolic bruit that radiates to the flank. The history may include atherosclerosis, anomalies of the renal arteries, recent trauma, or renal tumor.

Thyrotoxicosis (thyroid storm). The patient will experience a sudden rise in systolic blood pressure accompanied by widened pulse pressure, tachycardia, bounding pulse, pulsations in the capillary nail beds, and palpitations. Other findings may include exophthalmos, an enlarged thyroid gland, signs of dehydration (from episodes of diarrhea), a temperature above 100° F (37.8° C), and warm, moist skin. The patient may appear nervous and emotionally unstable, displaying occasional outbursts or even psychotic behavior. You may also note heat intolerance, exertional dyspnea and, in women, a history of decreased or absent menses. If the patient has latent hyperthyroidism, the history may include excessive dietary intake of iodine and repeated episodes of the symptoms following stressful conditions such as surgery, infections, pregnancy, or diabetic ketoacidosis.

Other causes

Certain causes of hypertension may not require immediate intervention.

Disorders. Hypertension may occur with congenital cardiac anomalies, mercury poisoning, and any condition that increases fluid volume.

Drugs. Among medications that can cause elevated blood pressure are central nervous system stimulants, sympathomimetics, corticosteroids, and oral contraceptives. Cocaine use can also raise blood pressure.

Hyperthermia

The term hyperthermia means an elevation of the core body temperature above normal. A temperature between 99° and 102° F (37.2° and 38.9° C) is considered mild hyperthermia; a temperature between 102° and 105° F (38.9° and 40.6° C), moderate hyperthermia. A temperature of 105° F (40.6° C) or above is considered critical hyperthermia and represents an emergency — particularly if the temperature rises rapidly or stays elevated for a prolonged period (see *Managing critical hyperthermia*). If a pa-

EMERGENCY INTERVENTION

Managing critical hyperthermia

If your patient's temperature is greater than 105° F (40.6° C), take his other vital signs and assess his level of consciousness before you notify the doctor. Then intervene as follows:
• Administer antipyretic drugs as ordered to lower the sensitivity of the patient's heat-regulation center and to produce diaphoresis.
• Begin rapid cooling measures. Apply ice packs to the patient's axillae and groin. Also, give him tepid sponge baths, or apply a hypothermia blanket.
• Give fluids, unless contraindicated. For an adult, fluid intake should be at least 2,500 to 3,000 ml. The patient may need a nasogastric tube, so cool fluids can be given to bring his temperature down quickly.
• Remember that these methods may evoke a hypothermic response. To prevent this, monitor the patient's core temperature. Watch for chills and shivering and adjust your interventions accordingly.

How hyperthermia develops

Body temperature is regulated by the hypothalamic thermostat, which has a specific set point under normal conditions. Hyperthermia can result from an adjustment of this set point or from an abnormality in the thermoregulatory system itself. This flowchart shows the events that can trigger these two mechanisms.

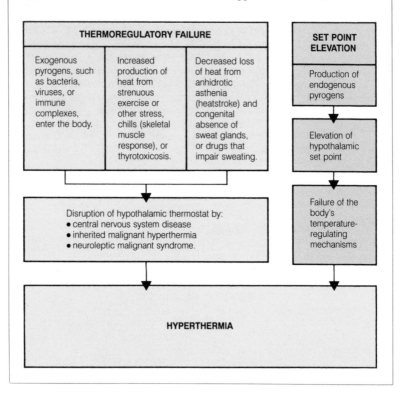

tient's core body temperature increases 2° F (1° C) every 15 minutes, the condition is called malignant hyperthermia. This occurs in persons who have an inherited predisposition to the condition.

Hyperthermia usually results from one or more pathophysiologic mechanisms (see *How hyperthermia develops*). One mechanism triggering hyperthermia is a resetting of the hypothalamic thermoregulatory control. In response to fever, for example, the core temperature is reset at a higher than normal level.

Another mechanism involves damage to the hypothalamic regulatory center itself. Here, the core temperature rises rapidly. This elevation may be temporary (if, for example, it's caused by heatstroke) or permanent (as may happen with head trauma or cerebral hemorrhage). A permanent increase is fatal.

History questions

Explore the patient's problem by asking appropriate questions from this section. If the patient requires emergency intervention, continue collecting the history as you intervene or when he's stable.

• Find out how long the patient has had a fever and whether it started suddenly or gradually. Have him describe its pattern: Did the temperature rise progressively? Rise and disappear, then reappear?

• Ask the patient about any accompanying symptoms, such as chills, headache, fatigue, diarrhea, or pain.

• Has he had an infection recently? Or can he recall a recent exposure to an infectious organism? Perhaps he traveled to an endemic area, or maybe he came in contact with insect or animal vectors, such as ticks carrying Rocky Mountain spotted fever.

• Ask the patient if he's been exposed to high temperatures for a prolonged period. Specifically, ask about his work environment. If he works in a warm environment, how much water does he drink while at work?

• Has the patient experienced unusual physical or emotional stress recently? Ask if he's had any burns or trauma, undergone surgery under general anesthesia, or received a blood transfusion.

• Does the patient have a history of endocrine dysfunction or malignant hypertension? Is he taking thyroid medication? If so, determine whether he's taking it as ordered. What about other medications that can disrupt thermoregulatory function (such as salicylates) or those

that impair sweating (such as antibiotics, anticholinergics, monoamine oxidase (MAO) inhibitors, or phenytoin)?

• Find out if the patient takes a drug with the potential for abuse—amphetamines or antidepressants, for instance. Did he poison himself accidentally or attempt suicide?

Physical examination

Base your assessment of the patient on the health history information you've collected. Be sure to auscultate the abdomen before palpating and percussing it. Using this sequence ensures that you don't affect the frequency or intensity of bowel sounds before you assess them.

Inspection. Note the rate and depth of the patient's breathing and any changes from normal respiratory patterns. Inspect skin color and temperature. Then check for skin turgor and diaphoresis.

Observe the patient's arms and legs for needle marks. Also, check him for signs of trauma—bruises and lacerations—and lesions that may indicate underlying disease. Is he shivering or is his face flushed? Inspect his oral mucosa for lesions and signs of dehydration. Look for drainage from the ears or nose.

After assessing his mental status, observe for a decline in his level of consciousness (LOC). Be alert, too, for signs of malaise, fatigue, restlessness, or anxiety. Observe his motor activity for possible muscle tremors, twitching, and rigidity.

Auscultation. Listen to all lung fields for adventitious sounds, especially rhonchi, crackles, or diminished breath sounds. As you auscultate the abdomen for bowel sounds, note characteristics such as pitch. If possible, take blood pressure readings with the patient both supine and sitting to detect orthostatic changes. Monitor his blood pressure and pulse pressure.

Palpation. Note the rate, rhythm, and intensity of the patient's peripheral pulses. As you palpate the abdominal quadrants, check for masses, and note any pain, tenderness, rigidity, or guarding. Gently palpate the scalp for crepitus or tenderness, and carefully feel the neck for thyroid enlargement or masses. Keep in mind that palpating the thyroid of a person with hyperthyroidism can induce thyrotoxicosis.

Percussion. Listen for increased dullness or hyperresonance as you percuss the lung fields and abdominal quadrants. Check the deep tendon reflexes, noting any abnormal responses.

Life-threatening causes

Your assessment may lead you to suspect one or more of the following.

Infectious and inflammatory disorders. Depending on the specific disorder, the temperature elevation may be insidious or abrupt. It can be a prodromal symptom and is often accompanied by chills, goosebumps, generalized symptoms of fatigue, headache, weakness, anorexia, malaise, and possibly pain. If the temperature is high, you may find that the patient, particularly an elderly person, is disoriented or delirious. Other associated signs and symptoms depend on the disease and can involve any system. The patient's history may include exposure to an infectious agent, travel to an endemic area, or exposure to the animal or insect vector of an infec-

tious organism. Or his recent history may include a blood transfusion, surgery, trauma, or burns.

Malignant hyperthermia. Rapid temperature increases occur at a rate of about 2° F (1° C) every 15 minutes to as high as 109.4° F (43° C). Usually, the rise is preceded by skeletal muscle rigidity, cardiac dysrhythmia, tachycardia, and tachypnea. The patient's history will include exposure to inhalant anesthetics, particularly halothane, or muscle relaxants, particularly succinylcholine, which can trigger malignant hyperthermia in patients with the inherited trait. The patient may not know he has the trait. Other precipitating factors in susceptible persons include trauma, exercise, exposure to high environmental temperatures, and infection.

Neuroleptic malignant syndrome. This syndrome is marked by an explosive onset of hyperthermia accompanied by muscle rigidity, altered LOC, cardiac dysrhythmias, tachycardia, wide fluctuations in blood pressure, postural instability, dyspnea, and tachypnea. The patient's history will include use of neuroleptic drugs such as haloperidol, chlorpromazine, thioridazine, or thiothixene.

Thermoregulatory dysfunction. With this disorder, the patient's temperature rises suddenly and rapidly. The temperature then stays at 105° to 107° F (40.6° to 41.7° C). You may note vomiting, anhidrosis, hot flushed skin, and a decreased LOC. The patient may also have such related cardiovascular effects as tachycardia, tachypnea, or hypotension. Other findings may include mottled cyanosis if the patient has malignant hyperthermia; diarrhea if he's experiencing a thyroid storm; ominous signs of increased intracranial pressure (decreased LOC with bradycardia, widened pulse pressure, and increased systolic pressure) when the problem is central nervous system trauma or hemorrhage. Heatstroke, brain stem compression (from head trauma, cerebral hemorrhage, or ischemia), and thyroid storm are common causes of thermoregulatory dysfunction. Toxic doses of amphetamines or salicylates will also disrupt the thermoregulatory centers. The patient's history will usually indicate prolonged exposure to conditions of high temperature and humidity, recent head trauma, thyroid dysfunction, substance abuse, or suspected accidental poisoning.

Other causes
Hyperthermia also results from certain causes that may not require immediate intervention.

Disorders. Impaired heat dissipation may result in hyperthermia. This occurs with severe dehydration, in which reduced sweat production decreases heat loss by evaporation. It also occurs when the environmental temperature is high, and the body can't get rid of heat as fast as it's being received.

Drugs. Hyperthermia can result from use of tricyclic antidepressants and drugs that impair sweating such as anticholinergics, phenothiazines, and MAO inhibitors. A rise in temperature can represent a hypersensitivity reaction to certain drugs and may occur several weeks after taking them.

Hypotension

The term hypotension refers to blood pressure that's too low to allow normal perfusion or oxygenation. Because normal blood pressure varies, low blood pressure can be determined only by comparing a current pressure reading with the patient's baseline reading. Typically, a reading below 90/60 mm Hg or a drop of 30 mm Hg from the baseline is considered hypotension. Children under age 12 normally have lower blood pressure (see *Guide to pediatric blood pressure*).

Low blood pressure can reflect an expanded intravascular space and normal intravascular volume (as

Guide to pediatric blood pressure

AGE	NORMAL SYSTOLIC PRESSURE	NORMAL DIASTOLIC PRESSURE
Birth to 3 months	40 to 80 mm Hg	Not detectable
3 months to 1 year	80 to 100 mm Hg	Not detectable
1 to 4 years	100 to 108 mm Hg	60 mm Hg
4 to 12 years	For every year, add 2 mm Hg to 100 mm Hg	60 to 70 mm Hg

with vasodilation), a reduced intravascular volume (as with dehydration or hemorrhage), or a decreased cardiac output (as with impaired myocardial contractility). Because the body's pressure-regulating mechanisms are complex and interrelated, several factors usually contribute to low blood pressure.

History questions

Explore the patient's problem by asking appropriate questions from this section.

• Ask the patient if he's been experiencing unusual fatigue, weakness, dizziness, or fainting. If so, were these symptoms related to activity or changes in position? Have him describe any headaches as specifically as possible. Is he bleeding — either externally or internally? Does he have tissue damage or burns?

• Does the patient have chest or abdominal pain or difficulty breathing? Is the pain intermittent or constant? Does it radiate?

• Ask if he has any bowel or bladder difficulty, such as incontinence, anuria, or oliguria. Is he excessively thirsty? Does he have polyuria?

• Does he have any associated motor dysfunction — such as seizures or tremors — or feelings of restlessness or anxiety?

• Does he have a history of low blood pressure and has he had similar episodes? Is he supposed to take medication for these episodes? Does he take it as prescribed?

• Has the patient been exposed to a common allergen or recently been stung by an insect, particularly a bee? Has he changed his diet or physical environment?

• Has he recently had any infections, periods of nausea, vomiting, or diarrhea? Has he lost weight? Does he have a nasogastric tube in place that's draining fluid? If you suspect fluid loss, try to determine the source and estimate the volume lost.

• Has he suffered recent trauma — such as blunt chest trauma or spinal cord injury? What about a recent cardiac arrest for which he received closed-chest cardiac massage?

• Determine if the patient's history includes cardiac, adrenal, or GI disease; diabetes mellitus; deep vein thrombosis; exposure to noxious stimuli; or alcoholism.

• Has the patient undergone any recent invasive procedures, surgery, or immunosuppressive therapy that could predispose him to infection? What about diagnostic tests that use contrast media or histamine, such as X-rays or a gastric acid stimulation test?

• Note any medications the patient is taking. Remember that penicillins and sulfonamides are associated with anaphylaxis; aspirin and some other drugs can cause bleeding; diuretics can cause excessive fluid loss; and beta blockers can lower blood pressure or cause congestive heart failure.

Physical examination

Base your assessment of the patient on the health history information you've collected.

Inspection. Examine the patient's skin for pallor, flushing, cyanosis, poor turgor, hyperpigmentation, and diaphoresis. Note any areas of erythema or skin eruptions that may indicate an allergic reaction. Also, look for bruising (particularly on the abdomen and chest), bleeding, or edema. Then test capillary refill time. To check for dehydration, inspect the patient's mucous membranes. Note any jugular vein distention.

Assess the patient's level of consciousness (LOC), and watch for any deterioration or seizures. Observe his breathing, noting the rate and depth. Does he have difficulty breathing? Do you see any abnormal patterns such as Cheyne-Stokes or Kussmaul's respirations? Monitor urine output for oliguria or anuria.

Palpation. Note the rate, rhythm, and intensity of the peripheral pulses. Then check the limbs and sacral area for edema. Also, feel the skin temperature of the arms and legs. Palpate for hepatomegaly.

Percussion. Note any tenderness or rigidity as you percuss the abdomen.

Auscultation. Monitor the patient's blood pressure and pulse pressure (see *Determining blood pressure accurately*, page 108). If your patient has a history of cardiac disease, be sure to obtain blood pressure readings from both arms. If he reports weakness or fainting after changing positions, take blood pressure readings with him supine, sitting, and standing. Compare the readings. If systolic or diastolic pressure drops 10 mm Hg or more when the patient changes position, he has orthostatic hypotension.

Note pulsus paradoxus, an accentuated fall in systolic pressure during inspiration. Listen for abnormal heart rhythms and sounds, such as gallops or murmurs. Auscultate for bradycardia or tachycardia.

Auscultate the lungs for abnormal breath sounds (diminished sounds, crackles, wheezes, or pleural friction rubs) or rhythms (agonal respirations). Note bradypnea or tachypnea. Listen, too, for abnormal bowel sounds.

Life-threatening causes

Your assessment may lead you to suspect one or more of the following.

Acute adrenal failure. A sudden, unexpected hypotensive episode that occurs during a serious illness, after minor trauma, or during the early postoperative period suggests acute adrenal failure. Sometimes the hypotension develops only after a long, progressive, destructive process. In this case, the hypotension is usually orthostatic. Associated signs and symptoms include fatigue, progressive weakness, irritability, headache, severe abdominal discomfort or pain, anorexia, weight loss, nausea and vomiting, diarrhea, fever, and oliguria. You'll find the patient's pulse rapid and thready, his skin cool and clammy, and his arms and legs flaccid. If the patient has chronic adrenocortical hypofunction, you may observe hyperpigmentation of the skin and mucous membranes. The patient's history may include preexisting adrenal disease and poor compliance with his medical regimen. His history may also include either recent trauma or stress that precipitated a crisis.

Anaphylactic shock. You'll note a dramatic fall in blood pressure and a narrowed pulse pressure (the difference between the systolic and diastolic pressures) in a patient with this disorder. Usually, these changes follow extreme anxiety, restlessness, a feeling of doom, intense itching (especially of the hands and feet), and a pounding headache. Symptoms typically begin within seconds or minutes of exposure to an allergen, but delayed reactions of up to 24 hours can occur. Later signs and symptoms may include flushing, cardiac dysrhythmias, weak and rapid pulse, seizures,

Determining blood pressure accurately

When you take the patient's blood pressure, begin by applying the cuff properly, as shown. Then, be alert for the common pitfalls described below.

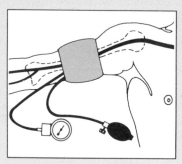

Wrong-sized cuff
Select the appropriate-sized cuff for the patient. This ensures that adequate pressure is applied to compress the brachial artery during cuff inflation. If the cuff bladder is too narrow, the reading will be falsely high. If it's too wide, the reading will be falsely low. The cuff bladder width should be about 40% of the circumference of the midpoint of the arm; bladder length should be twice the width. If the arm circumference is less than 13″ (33 cm), select a regular-sized cuff; if it's between 13″ and 16″ (33 and 41 cm), a large-sized cuff; if it's more than 16″, a thigh cuff. Pediatric cuffs are also available.

Loosely wrapped cuff
This reduces the cuff's effective width. Tighten the cuff to avoid a falsely elevated reading.

Poorly timed measurement
Don't take the blood pressure if the patient appears anxious or has just eaten or ambulated; you'll get a falsely high reading.

Incorrect arm position
Keep the patient's arm level with his heart to avoid a falsely low reading.

Cuff overinflation
Overinflation can cause venospasm or pain, leading to a falsely high reading.

Slow cuff deflation
This causes venous congestion in the extremity. Don't deflate the cuff more slowly than 2 mm Hg/heartbeat or you'll get a falsely high reading.

Unnoted auscultatory gap
In an auscultatory gap, sound fades out for 10 to 15 mm Hg, then returns. To avoid missing the top Korotkoff's sound, first estimate systolic pressure by palpation. Then inflate the cuff rapidly—at a rate of 2 to 3 mm Hg/second—to about 30 mm Hg above the palpable systolic pressure.

Inaudible feeble sounds
Before you reinflate the cuff, have the patient raise his arm to reduce venous pressure and amplify low volume sounds. After inflating the cuff, lower his arm. Then deflate the cuff and listen. Or, with the patient's arm at heart level, inflate the cuff and tell him to make a fist. Have him rapidly open and close his hand 10 times before you begin to deflate the cuff. Then listen. Document that the blood pressure reading was augmented.

Wrong reading level
Read the mercury column at eye level. If the column is below your eye level, you may record a falsely low reading; if it's above your eye level, a falsely high reading.

Tilted mercury column
Keep the mercury column vertical to avoid a falsely high reading.

coughing, sneezing, difficulty breathing, nasal congestion, stridor and hoarseness from laryngeal edema, chest or throat tightness, nausea, abdominal cramps, and fecal and urinary incontinence. The patient may have a known allergy or a family history of allergies. His recent history will include exposure to an allergen, especially bee venom or a drug such as a penicillin or sulfonamide (see *Identifying causes of shock*, page 110).

Cardiac contusion. If a patient has suffered recent blunt chest trauma, his low blood pressure will be accompanied by tachycardia, chest pain unrelieved by coronary vasodilator drugs, and dyspnea. The chest pain will be excruciating but intermittent. It may radiate to the neck, jaw, or arm. When you examine the patient, you may see bruises on the chest and abdomen.

Cardiac dysrhythmias. In patients with dysrhythmias, low blood pressure may alternate with normal readings. This may be accompanied by symptoms that reflect the type and severity of the underlying problem. Thus, you may find generalized weak pulses, cool and clammy skin, dizziness, light-headedness, weakness, fatigue, chest pain, decreased LOC, and palpitations. Auscultation typically will reveal a pulse greater than 100 beats/minute or less than 60 beats/minute or an irregular rhythm. The patient's history may indicate cardiac disease.

Cardiac tamponade. Hypotension, narrowed pulse pressure, neck vein distention, and muffled heart sounds are the classic signs of cardiac tamponade. This disorder also produces tachycardia, pulsus paradoxus, dyspnea, Kussmaul's respirations, and cyanosis. The patient's history may include recent chest trauma, pericarditis, myocardial infarction (MI), fever, malaise, or chronic tamponade.

Cardiogenic shock. With this disorder, you'll note a drop in systolic pressure to less than 80 mm Hg or to 30 mm Hg less than the patient's baseline. Accompanying signs include narrowed pulse pressure, diminished Korotkoff's sounds, peripheral cyanosis, and pale, cool, clammy skin. Cardiogenic shock also causes restlessness and anxiety, which may progress to disorientation and confusion. Associated signs and symptoms include anginal pain, dyspnea, neck vein distention, oliguria, and a weak, rapid pulse. On auscultation, you may detect tachypnea, tachycardia, faint heart sounds, ventricular gallop, and a systolic murmur. The patient's history may include disorders that cause left ventricular dysfunction.

Congestive heart failure. Because of pump failure, blood pressure readings may fluctuate between normal and low in patients with congestive heart failure (CHF). However, a precipitous drop in blood pressure may be a harbinger of cardiogenic shock. Your auscultation will indicate ventricular gallop, tachycardia, bilateral crackles, and tachypnea. You may also find dependent edema, jugular vein distention, prolonged capillary refill time (greater than 2 seconds), and hepatomegaly. The patient's history may reveal dyspnea with an abrupt or gradual onset, fatigue, weight gain, pallor or cyanosis, diaphoresis, and anxiety. You may also learn that the patient isn't complying with a prescribed regimen for heart disease. His medication history may include

Identifying causes of shock

Shock may result from many causes. Use this quick-reference list to help identify its common causes.

Anaphylactic shock
- Anesthetics (cocaine, lidocaine, procaine, thiopental)
- Antibiotics (penicillin, penicillin analogs, cephalosporins, tetracyclines, erythromycin, streptomycin)
- Blood, blood products, and vaccines (transfusions of red cells, white cells, and platelets; gamma globulin; rabies, tetanus, and diphtheria antitoxins)
- Diagnostic contrast media containing iodine
- Foods and dyes (eggs, milk, nuts, peanuts, soybeans, kidney beans, shellfish, fruits [especially strawberries], tartrazine [FD&C yellow dye No. 5])
- Hormones (insulin, pituitary extract, adrenocorticotropic hormone)
- Narcotic analgesics (morphine, codeine, meprobamate)
- Nonsteroidal anti-inflammatory agents (salicylates, aminopyrine, indomethacin)
- Other drugs (iodides, thiazide diuretics, protamine, chlorpropamide, parenteral iron)
- Pollens (ragweed, grasses)
- Venoms (bee, wasp, hornet, yellow jacket, spider, snake, jellyfish)

Cardiogenic shock
- Decreased left ventricular function (myocardial ischemia or infarction, valvular disease, cardiac tamponade, open-heart surgery, cardiomyopathy)
- Medications (inotropic drugs, vasodilators, calcium channel blockers)

Hypovolemic shock
- Internal fluid loss (third-space shifting; fluid leakage into intestinal lumen; long-bone fracture; internal hemorrhage—hemorrhagic pancreatitis, hemothorax, ruptured spleen)
- External fluid loss (blood loss from multiple trauma, GI hemorrhage, surgery, or bleeding disorder; plasma loss from burn or large exudative lesions; body fluid loss from nasogastric suctioning, fistulas, vomiting, diarrhea, excessive diuretic use, diabetes mellitus or insipidus, or Addison's disease)

Neurogenic shock
- Upper spinal-cord injury or disease
- High spinal anesthesia
- Vasomotor center depression
- Exposure to noxious stimuli
- Massive head injury (rare)

Septic shock
- Burns
- Chronic disorders (hepatic dysfunction, cardiac disease, renal disease, diabetes mellitus, alcoholism)
- Excessive antibiotic use
- Immunosuppression (neoplastic disorders, radiation therapy, cytotoxic drug therapy, corticosteroid therapy, immunosuppressive drug therapy)
- Invasive procedures or devices (I.V. lines, central catheters)
- Malnutrition
- Stress
- Surgical procedures and wounds

angiotensin-converting enzyme inhibitors, beta blockers, corticosteroids, nonsteroidal anti-inflammatory drugs, antihypertensives, antiarrhythmics, carbamazepine, recombinant interferon alpha-2a, or recombinant interleukin-2.

Diabetic ketoacidosis. If low blood pressure accompanies facial flushing, tachycardia, and decreased pulse pressure, the cause may be osmotic diuresis and dehydration from diabetic ketoacidosis. Loss of sodium and extracellular fluid with this condition can also produce abdominal pain, nausea, vomiting, Kussmaul's respirations, seizures, and stupor that may progress to coma. The patient may have experienced polydipsia, polyuria, polyphagia, weight loss, and weakness for several days. His history may include diabetes mellitus.

Hyperosmolar hyperglycemic nonketotic coma. In this disorder, the patient's blood pressure decreases, sometimes dramatically, when osmotic diuresis causes significant fluid loss. Typically, the patient has had polyuria, polydipsia, weight loss, fever, tachycardia, poor skin turgor, shallow respirations, soft eyeballs, and deteriorating mental status over several days or weeks. The mental changes may range from confusion to coma and occasionally include generalized motor seizures. The patient's history may reveal Type II diabetes mellitus and, perhaps, noncompliance with his medication or dietary regimen.

Hypovolemic shock. In this disorder, systolic pressure drops to less than 80 mm Hg or to 30 mm Hg less than the patient's baseline. Accompanying signs and symptoms include orthostatic pressure changes, diminished Korotkoff's sounds, narrowed pulse pressure, tachypnea and tachycardia that increase as blood volume decreases, and a weak and occasionally irregular pulse. You may also note prolonged capillary refill time (greater than 2 seconds), hypothermia, light-headedness, irritability, diaphoresis, extreme thirst, oliguria, angina (if the patient has coronary artery disease), and mental changes such as confusion, disorientation, restlessness, and anxiety. Peripheral vasoconstriction causes cyanosis of the limbs and pale, cool, clammy skin. The patient's history will reveal a source of blood volume loss.

Myocardial infarction. Blood pressure may either rise or fall when an MI occurs. The disorder is characterized by crushing chest pain that may radiate to the jaw, shoulder, arm, or epigastrium. It's accompanied by dyspnea, anxiety, nausea, vomiting, weakness, diaphoresis, and cool, pale, or cyanotic skin. On auscultation, you may note an atrial gallop or murmur and, occasionally, an irregular pulse. The patient may have a history or family history of cardiac disease. He may report recent unusual stress or a life-style that includes excessive sodium and fat intake, lack of exercise, and smoking. His history may also reveal cocaine use, which can cause an MI.

Neurogenic shock. Hypotension and bradycardia are the cardinal signs of neurogenic shock, although in most cases the systolic pressure doesn't fall below 100 mm Hg. Vasodilation causes the relative hypovolemia that produces the symptoms. Vasodilation also keeps the skin warm, dry, and, sometimes, flushed. The patient's history will disclose a condition that can cause neurogenic shock.

Pulmonary embolism. Hypotension with narrowed pulse pressure and diminished Korotkoff's sounds occur in this disorder. Accompanying signs and symptoms include sudden chest pain, dyspnea, and cyanosis. You can usually hear crackles on auscultation, and you're likely to detect hepatomegaly. You may also note tachycardia, tachypnea, and neck vein distention. If a pulmonary infarction has developed, you'll note hemoptysis, severe pleuritic chest pain, pleural friction rub, and fever. The patient's history may include deep vein thrombosis, varicose veins, disorders that decrease cardiac output, or cardiac valvular disease. The history may also include a recent hospitalization, immobility, or prolonged surgical procedures.

Septic shock. In the late stage of septic shock, hypotension becomes severe, with blood pressure dropping to less than 80 mm Hg or 50 to 80 mm Hg less than the patient's baseline. Accompanying signs and symptoms may include a narrowed pulse pressure, tachycardia, dysrhythmias, a weak and thready pulse, decreased or absent peripheral pulses, rapid and shallow respirations, a decreased LOC possibly progressing to coma, pale skin, cyanotic limbs, and oliguria or anuria from decreased cardiac output. The patient's history may include conditions that predispose him to septic shock.

Other causes
Certain causes of hypotension may not require immediate intervention.

Diagnostic tests. The gastric acid stimulation test using histamine and X-ray studies using contrast media can cause blood pressure to drop by triggering allergic reactions.

Drugs. Antihypertensive drugs obviously can cause blood pressure to drop. So can beta blockers, calcium channel blockers, diuretics, and vasodilators. Low blood pressure can also be caused by general anesthetics, narcotic analgesics, monoamine oxidase inhibitors, antianxiety agents, tranquilizers, and most I.V. antiarrhythmics (especially bretylium tosylate).

Hypothermia

The term hypothermia means that the core body temperature is below normal 98.6° F (37° C). A temperature between 93° and 97° F (33.9° and 36.1° C) is classified as mild hypothermia; a temperature between 82° and 92° F (27.7° and 33.3° C), moderate hypothermia; a temperature between 62° and 81° F (16.7° and 27.2° C), deep hypothermia; and a temperature between 39° and 61° F (3.8° and 16.1° C), profound hypothermia.

Sometimes, hypothermia is induced deliberately, as with cardiovascular surgery and neurosurgery. Many times, it's accidental—for instance, when someone is exposed to cold temperatures or receives a rapid infusion of refrigerated blood (see *How to treat hypothermia*).

Whatever the cause, the result is the same. The person's core body temperature drops, cooling the brain and depressing the thermoregulatory center in the hypothalamus. When this happens, the ability to regulate body temperature is lost. Metabolic processes and nerve conduction slow progressively, resulting in coma and, eventually, respiratory and circulatory failure (see *Understanding the effects of hypothermia,* page 114). Elderly and debilitated people are especially susceptible to hypothermia.

History questions
Explore the patient's problem by asking appropriate questions from this section. If the patient requires emergency intervention, continue collecting the history as you intervene or when he's stable.
• Find out if the patient has recently

been exposed to cold temperatures or immersed in cold water. If so, how long was he exposed?

• Determine if the patient has adequate heat in his home. Or is he homeless and sleeping outside?

• Verify the patient's age.

• Find out if he's recently undergone major surgery or surgery that required cooling of his body. Has he recently received a transfusion of blood that may have been administered while still cold?

• Does the patient's history include thyroid, adrenal, liver, or cerebrovascular disease? How about diabetes mellitus?

• Has he ingested any substances that could induce hypothermia, such as alcohol or barbiturates?

Physical examination

Base your assessment of the patient on the health history information you've collected.

Inspection. Observe the patient's skin color and check his capillary refill time. If he's experienced trauma, check the skin for bruises, lacerations, and bleeding. Note the rate and depth of his breathing and any abnormal respiratory patterns. Does he have difficulty breathing? Inspect his oral mucosa for signs of cyanosis. Look for abdominal distention suggesting ascites.

Palpation. Note the rate, rhythm, and intensity of the peripheral pulses. If the patient has experienced trauma, palpate his abdomen for tenderness and guarding. Gently feel his scalp for crepitus and tenderness. Then carefully palpate the long bones to detect any fractures. If fractures have been ruled out, slowly move the patient's arms and legs through a small range of motion to detect any muscle stiffness.

EMERGENCY INTERVENTION

How to treat hypothermia

The earlier you recognize hypothermia, the more likely you'll be successful in treating it. You can expect to find hypothermia in patients who fall into one of these high-risk groups:

• elderly people (because of inadequate heating and chronic disease)

• alcoholics and homeless people who fall asleep outdoors

• hikers and campers in mountainous areas.

Treating hypothermia consists of rewarming, but you have to do this carefully to prevent further damage to your patient. You can use active or passive measures.

Active external rewarming can be achieved by such measures as immersing the patient in warm water or applying electric blankets or heatingpads. The disadvantage of this method is that it may increase hypotension and hypovolemia by dilating the peripheral blood vessels in skin and muscle before it affects the central vessels of the brain, heart, and kidneys.

Other active rewarming alternatives are considered aggressive measures and appropriate only for patients who have temperatures below 85° F (29.4°) or those who are comatose. These invasive techniques include peritoneal dialysis, hemodialysis, intragastric lavage with warm fluids, and inhalation warming.

Passive rewarming means simply removing the patient from the cold environment and wrapping him in something warm and dry—such as a blanket. This can be done while you're waiting for transport to the hospital. If your patient is extremely hypothermic, you can speed up the rewarming process by removing his clothing and wrapping him in the blanket with another person. This allows for passive transfer of normal body heat.

Understanding the effects of hypothermia

The effects of hypothermia depend on its severity, as this flowchart shows.

MILD HYPOTHERMIA

- Increased shivering
- Altered mentation
- Worsened cardiac dysrhythmias (due to altered electrodynamics)

MODERATE HYPOTHERMIA

- Decreased pancreatic activity
- Body metabolism decreased by 50%
- Atrial dysrhythmias
- Heart rate lowered by 50%
- Pupils nonreactive to light
- Confusion

DEEP HYPOTHERMIA

- Possible circulatory arrest
- High risk for ventricular fibrillation
- Thermoregulatory centers inactivated
- Muscle reflexes absent
- Respiratory arrest imminent

PROFOUND HYPOTHERMIA

- Survival unlikely

Percussion. Listen for hyperresonance and dullness in the lungs and abdomen. Percuss the deep tendon reflexes and note any abnormalities.

Auscultation. Check all lung fields for adventitious or diminished breath sounds. Then listen to the entire abdomen to determine the characteristics of the patient's bowel sounds. Monitor his blood pressure and pulse pressure.

Life-threatening cause
Your assessment may lead you to suspect this disorder.

Prolonged exposure to extremely low temperatures. The patient will have deep or profound hypothermia accompanied by lethargy or coma, depressed respiratory rate and depth, bradycardia, and muscle stiffness. He may have been exposed to an extremely low temperature with an excessive wind chill factor. If the patient is elderly or debilitated, he may have been exposed to a low (but not necessarily extremely low) room temperature. Your patient may also have received a transfusion of chilled blood products.

Other causes
Hypothermia also results from certain causes that may not require immediate intervention.

Disorders. Hypothyroidism, hypoadrenalism, hypopituitarism, diabetes mellitus, advanced cirrhosis, and stroke can cause hypothermia.

Drugs. Alcohol ingestion and an overdose of barbiturates can induce mild to moderate hypothermia as a result of vasodilation, lowered metabolism, and central nervous system effects.

Level of consciousness, decreased

Because level of consciousness (LOC) is based on a subjective evaluation of the patient's behavior and appearance, it can be difficult to define. But intuitively we know that a conscious person is aware of his surroundings and interacts with his environment. Any behavior showing diminished awareness or interaction is defined as a decrease in the LOC.

To assess consciousness, you need to evaluate two components: the level of *content*, which includes determining how well the patient is using the higher mental functions of the brain, and the level of *arousal*, which means determining his state of wakefulness. Alterations in the level of arousal may be described as confusion, delirium, obtundation, stupor, or coma.

The reticular activating system (RAS) — an intricate network of neurons whose axons extend from the brain stem, thalamus, and hypothalamus to the cerebral cortex — controls consciousness. A disturbance in any part of this integrated system impairs the communication that makes consciousness possible. A patient's LOC can be affected by an impairment in the cerebral hemispheres or by dysfunction of the RAS caused by tissue destruction from hemorrhage. Ketones, bacteria, viruses, and other toxic endogenous or exogenous substances can also induce changes in consciousness.

Cerebral dysfunction usually produces the least dramatic decrease in LOC. By contrast, dysfunction of the RAS produces the most dramatic decrease in a patient's LOC — coma.

A wide spectrum of subtle and not-so-subtle changes can cause diminished consciousness, and the same change in LOC can result from either a benign or an ominous condition. For instance, inattentiveness may be brought on by simple fatigue or by life-threatening increased intracranial pressure (ICP). Consciousness can deteriorate suddenly or gradually and remain altered temporarily or permanently. A marked decrease in the LOC, however, commonly signals a life-threatening situation (see *Case in point: When your patient is unconscious*, page 116).

History questions

Explore the patient's problem by asking appropriate questions from this section. Remember, though, a change in his LOC may impair his ability to answer history questions accurately. So you may need to get information from a family member or someone who brought him to the hospital. If emergency treatment is needed, continue asking questions as you intervene.

• When did the patient or family first notice a change in behavior, personality, memory, temperament, or level of arousal? How long after the precipitating event did the change occur? Did the change occur suddenly or gradually? Since the change, has the patient's behavior remained the same, deteriorated, or improved? Ask the patient, family, or witness to describe the precipitating event and the behavior change in detail.

• Did the patient complain of headache, dizziness, nausea, vomiting, visual disturbances, or any other problems before his LOC declined? Investigate any symptoms that

EMERGENCY INTERVENTION

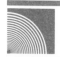

Case in point: When your patient is unconscious

When a patient exhibits a sign or symptom that could indicate an emergency, you need to perform a quick, thorough assessment. That way, you can determine if his condition is truly life-threatening and how to intervene.

Consider the case of Greg Lane, age 19, who's brought to the emergency department unconscious. His friends tell you that he had a seizure before he became unconscious.

Assessing the danger
You quickly examine Greg and find that his respiratory rate is 6 breaths/minute; his pulse rate, 160 beats/minute; and his blood pressure, 150/90 mm Hg. He doesn't respond to verbal stimuli, and his pupils are dilated and react sluggishly to light. You note that he has good skin turgor and that his breath smells normal. During your inspection, you don't see any obvious head or body injuries.

Because the patient is unresponsive and has dilated pupils and a low respiratory rate, the doctor intubates him. You use manual artificial ventilation until the ventilator is set up. In case emergency medications are necessary, an I.V. line is inserted and dextrose 5% in water administered.

Zeroing in on the cause
As you're assessing Greg, you ask his friends some health history questions.

Although they don't know much about Greg's past, they were with him when he lost consciousness. They tell you Greg was complaining of chest pain just before the seizure. Based on this information, Greg is placed on a cardiac monitor, which shows sinus tachycardia.

His friends tell you Greg doesn't have any conditions such as diabetes. But when you ask them if he takes any medications, they admit that he'd been smoking cocaine before the chest pain began.

Because there's no antidote for cocaine toxicity, you continuously monitor Greg for complications, such as cardiac dysrhythmias, cardiac arrest, hypothermia, hypertension, and seizures. The doctor orders toxicology studies to confirm that cocaine precipitated the symptoms. He also orders studies to rule out myocardial infarction and head injury.

Evaluating your care
Your quick assessment of Greg enabled you to determine that his primary sign really did indicate a life-threatening condition. And your systematic approach allowed you to uncover the underlying cause of Greg's unconsciousness. Thus, you were able to intervene appropriately by closely monitoring Greg's condition until he recovered.

the patient has experienced. If he's been vomiting, is it projectile, forceful, or persistent? If he has a headache, have him describe the pain. Is it excruciating? Is it localized? Does it get worse when he strains during a bowel movement?
• What about diarrhea, abdominal pain, fever, anorexia, seizures, progressive weakness, back or leg

pain, polydipsia, polyuria, polyphagia, photophobia, muscle cramps, or urinary incontinence?
• Has the patient had a traumatic head injury or been involved in a motor vehicle accident? Was he recently exposed to extremely cold or hot temperatures?
• Has the patient been exposed to any viruses or bacteria that are

known to cause encephalitis or meningitis? Does the patient have, or has he recently had, influenza, chicken pox, or a middle ear, sinus, or mastoid infection? Did he receive any vaccinations recently? Has he had recent dental work?

• Does the patient have any history of neurologic, cardiovascular, renal, hematologic, endocrine, or liver disorders? Does he have any disease or condition that would predispose him to a shock state — severe infection, severe cardiac disease, or spinal cord injury, for example? How about risk factors that could predispose him to cardiovascular disease — hypertension, a stressful life-style, smoking, or excessive caffeine intake?

• Does the patient abuse drugs or alcohol? If so, which ones and how frequently?

• If the patient is pregnant, does she have pregnancy-induced hypertension, or has she had it during previous pregnancies?

• Does the patient have a history of exposure to lead? Children who live in older homes may be at risk for ingestion of paint chips containing lead. With adults, check the occupational history for lead exposure.

• What medications is the patient taking? Has he recently received any sedatives or general anesthetics?

Physical examination
Base your assessment of the patient on the health history information you've collected.

Inspection. Evaluate the patient's LOC by addressing him in a normal voice and noting his response. Is it appropriate or abnormal? For instance, is his speech aphasic or slurred? Describe the patient's LOC

Describing LOC

The following list provides definitions of standard terms used to describe level of consciousness (LOC).

• **Awake:** The patient is alert and completely oriented. He responds to verbal and painful stimuli.
• **Sleep:** When awakened, the patient becomes alert and oriented. He responds to stimuli.
• **Confusion:** The patient has a short attention span and misinterprets information. He's disoriented to time, place, and person and has trouble following commands, but he still responds to stimuli.
• **Delirium:** The patient is disoriented, agitated, and perhaps combative. He may have hallucinations, and he responds to stimuli.
• **Obtundation:** When awakened, the patient remains drowsy, disoriented, and confused. He stays awake only if he's continuously stimulated.
• **Light stupor:** The patient doesn't respond to verbal stimuli, but he withdraws quickly and forcefully from moderate pain, which he can localize.
• **Deep stupor:** The patient responds only to a strong stimulus, which he can't localize. You may note decerebrate posture.
• **Coma:** The patient doesn't respond to any stimuli. His vital signs may be stable, however. You may note brain stem and spinal cord reflexes. An electroencephalogram (EEG) shows activity.
• **Cerebral death:** The patient's vital signs must be maintained artificially. He has no reflexes and no EEG activity. He doesn't respond to stimuli.

as precisely as possible, using standard terms accepted by your institution (see *Describing LOC*). Also, use the Glasgow Coma Scale to assess his LOC (see *Using the Glasgow Coma Scale*, page 118).

Using the Glasgow Coma Scale

Using subjective descriptions such as lethargic, obtunded, and stuporous can create problems when you're monitoring a patient's level of consciousness (LOC). Your evaluation and subjective descriptions can easily differ from another nurse's, causing subtle changes to be overlooked. That's where the Glasgow Coma Scale can help. It provides a more objective method of recording changes in LOC. The scale grades consciousness according to how well a patient responds in three specific areas—eye-opening, motor response, and verbal response.

The scale won't help you evaluate early changes in LOC, but it will help you detect life-threatening changes.

And although the scale doesn't determine a patient's exact LOC, it does provide an easy way to describe his overall neurologic status and to help detect and interpret changes from the baseline.

To use the Glasgow Coma Scale, test your patient's ability to respond to verbal, motor, and sensory stimulation. When determining the baseline, be sure to identify the type of stimulus (for example, nail bed pressure) and then use it consistently. A decreased score in one or more categories may signal an impending neurologic crisis. A patient scoring 7 or less is comatose and probably has severe neurologic damage.

TEST	REACTION	SCORE
Best eye-opening response	Open spontaneously	4
	Open to verbal command	3
	Open to pain	2
	No response	1
Best motor response	Obeys verbal command	6
	Localizes painful stimulus	5
	Flexion—withdrawal	4
	Flexion—abnormal (decorticate rigidity)	3
	Extension (decerebrate rigidity)	2
	No response	1
Best verbal response	Oriented and converses	5
	Disoriented and converses	4
	Inappropriate words	3
	Incomprehensible sounds	2
	No response	1
Total		3 to 15

This scale will help you standardize your evaluations when you're monitoring a patient's LOC.

Observe the patient's pupils for equality and reactivity to light. Also, note any dysconjugate movements, such as nystagmus. If you're certain the patient doesn't have a cervical injury, perform the doll's eye maneuver and observe eye movement. Inspect his head, face, and neck for signs of head trauma, including scalp lacerations, bleeding, drainage from the ears and nose, Battle's sign, raccoon eyes, and distended neck veins.

Observe the rate and depth of the patient's respirations. Note any difficulty breathing, and look for signs of dyspnea or abnormal patterns, such as Kussmaul's or Cheyne-Stokes respirations. Inspect the skin temperature and color, noting diaphoresis, cyanosis, hyperpigmentation, or edema. Check the mucous membranes of the mouth for hyperpigmentation or lead lines along the gums. Do you notice an abnormal breath odor, such as fruity breath or fetor hepaticus?

Observe all body movements. Watch for shivering, hemiparesis, tremor, and seizures. If the patient is able, have him walk as you observe for ataxia. Note any abnormal posturing, such as opisthotonos, or decorticate or decerebrate postures.

Inspect the patient's skin for needle marks, or "tracks," a sign of drug abuse. Then check his nares; if he snorts cocaine, he may have a perforated septum.

Palpation. As you palpate the patient's head, note any crepitus, which may indicate hematoma or fracture. If you suspect head trauma, carefully palpate the face to detect any facial fractures. Palpate the abdomen for areas of tenderness or pain, and check for hepatomegaly.

Test the patient's response to touch. Assess his response to painful stimuli by exerting firm pressure on his Achilles tendon or fingernails. You can classify his response as "obeys," "localizes," or "flexion withdrawal." Or use terminology accepted by your institution. If the patient doesn't have head or spinal cord trauma, gently move his head toward his chest. Note any resistance or decreased range of motion, indicating nuchal rigidity. Palpate the muscles of the arms and legs for decreased muscle tone, flaccidity, or rigidity. Flex and extend the limbs to determine if they're hypotonic or hypertonic. Palpate the peripheral pulses, noting rate, rhythm, and intensity.

Percussion. Check deep tendon reflexes for abnormal responses. Lightly percuss the abdomen for hyperresonance or flatness.

Auscultation. Listen to all lung fields for adventitious breath sounds, especially rhonchi and crackles. Auscultate the patient's heart rate and heart sounds. Note any murmurs or abnormal sounds. Monitor his blood pressure and check for widening or narrowing pulse pressure.

Life-threatening causes
Your assessment may lead you to suspect one or more of the following.

Acute adrenal failure. Changes in consciousness resulting from cytotoxic cerebral edema range from lethargy to coma. (For more information, see *What causes changes in LOC*, page 120.) These changes develop 8 to 12 hours after the on-

PATHOPHYSIOLOGY

What causes changes in LOC

Cerebral edema, an expansion of extravascular fluid compartments inside the brain, is the major cause of changes in level of consciousness (LOC). Such edema may result from head injury, cerebrovascular accident, a tumor or other intracranial lesion, or intracranial changes following brain surgery.

Cerebral edema can be vasogenic, cytotoxic, or ischemic. In vasogenic edema, vascular disruption increases vascular permeability, allowing dissolved particles and fluid to cross blood vessel membranes and leak into the white matter's extracellular space. When systemic blood pressure is elevated, this leakage of fluid worsens.

In cytotoxic edema, intracellular fluid expands in response to cellular toxins, affecting cells in both the white matter and gray matter of the brain.

Ischemic edema combines the characteristics of vasogenic and cytotoxic edema. As ischemic cells lose membrane integrity, fluid moves into the cells, causing intracellular edema. The process continues, with cells dying and extracellular edema developing.

In the list below, tissue impairment would be considered ischemic or vasogenic. The metabolic causes would be either ischemic or cytotoxic. Both the exogenous and endogenous causes are considered cytotoxic.

TISSUE IMPAIRMENT

Supratentorial lesions
Neoplasm, brain abscess, cerebral edema, encephalitis, intracerebral hemorrhage, subarachnoid hemorrhage, arterial and venous thrombosis, epidural hemorrhage, subdural hematoma, cerebral aneurysm, and cerebral contusion

Infratentorial lesions
Brain stem infarction, pontine hemorrhage, and cerebellar hemorrhage

METABOLIC CAUSES

Lack of energy substrate
Anoxia, hypoglycemia, ischemia, thiamine and niacin deficiency

EXOGENOUS CAUSES

Sedative drugs, alcohol, anticholinergics, cocaine, opiates, heavy metals, cyanide, methyl alcohol, ethylene glycol, and organic phosphates

ENDOGENOUS CAUSES

Organ system failure
Hepatic encephalopathy, diabetic ketoacidosis, hyperglycemic hyperosmolar nonketotic coma, hypertensive encephalopathy, and myxedema coma

Fluid and electrolyte imbalance
Dehydration, water intoxication, hyponatremia, hypernatremia, hypomagnesemia, hypermagnesemia, hypocalcemia, hypercalcemia, acidosis, and alkalosis

Toxins and infections
Sepsis, meningitis, and Reye's syndrome

Temperature regulation disturbance
Hypothermia and hyperthermia

set of adrenal failure and result from the lack of glucocorticoids and mineralocorticoids. Early associated findings depend on the speed of adrenal failure's onset. Sudden, unexpected hypotension occurring during a serious illness, after minor trauma, or during the early postoperative period suggests acute adrenal failure.

Sometimes adrenal failure occurs only after a long, progressive, destructive process. In this case, the patient will have orthostatic hypotension. Other early signs and symptoms include progressive weakness; irritability; anorexia; headache; diarrhea; abdominal pain; fever; rapid, thready pulse; oliguria; cool, clammy skin; flaccid arms and legs; nausea; and vomiting. A patient with chronic adrenocortical hypofunction may have hyperpigmented skin and mucous membranes. His medical history may include adrenal dysfunction or poor compliance with his medical regimen.

Brain abscess. Decreasing LOC, resulting from cytotoxic cerebral edema, will vary from drowsiness to deep stupor. The patient may also have a headache that intensifies over a few days, is aggravated by straining, localizes to a particular spot, and is accompanied by nausea, vomiting, and focal or generalized seizures. Depending on the abscess site, you may also observe aphasia, impaired visual acuity, hemiparesis, ataxia, tremor, and personality changes. Signs of infection, such as fever and pallor, usually develop late. In half the cases, however, the abscess remains encapsulated and these signs may not appear. The patient's history may include systemic, chronic middle ear, mastoid, or sinus infection; compound frac-

ture; osteomyelitis of the skull; or a penetrating head wound.

Cerebral aneurysm (ruptured). Ischemic cerebral edema may cause confusion, lethargy, stupor, or deep coma. The change in the patient's LOC occurs immediately after the abrupt onset of an excruciating headache accompanied by nausea and vomiting. Nuchal rigidity, leg and back pain, fever, restlessness, irritability, seizures, and blurred vision indicate meningeal irritation. Other findings depend on the site and severity of the hemorrhage. These may include hemiparesis, hemisensory deficit, dysphagia, downward or conjugate deviation of the eye toward the side of the lesion, gait ataxia, miotic but reactive pupils, and visual defects. The patient may have a history of hypertension or other cardiovascular disorders. His history may also include a stressful life-style, excessive caffeine intake, or smoking.

Cerebral contusion. Consciousness may decline gradually or suddenly from vasogenic cerebral edema, depending on the extent and severity of the contusion. The patient is usually unconscious for a prolonged period and may develop dilated, nonreactive pupils and decorticate or decerebrate posture. If he's conscious or recovers consciousness, he may be drowsy, confused, disoriented, agitated, or even violent. You may also find that the patient has blurred or double vision, fever, headache, pallor, diaphoresis, tachycardia, altered respirations, aphasia, or hemiparesis. Residual effects may include seizures, impaired mental status, emotional lability, slight hemiparesis, and vertigo. The patient's history may include head trauma within the past few days. In physical abuse cases, particularly child abuse, the true nature of the injury may not be revealed during the health history.

Diabetic ketoacidosis. A rapid decrease in LOC, ranging from lethargy to coma, results from cytotoxic cerebral edema. In many cases, this is preceded by polydipsia, polyphagia, polyuria, weakness, anorexia, abdominal pain, nausea, vomiting, orthostatic hypotension, fruity breath odor, Kussmaul's respirations, warm and dry skin, and a rapid, thready pulse. The patient may have a history of Type I diabetes mellitus, stress, and poor compliance with his medical regimen.

Encephalitis. With this disorder, consciousness will deteriorate over 48 hours, perhaps from lethargy to coma. This decreased LOC and the severe headache that accompanies it result from cytotoxic cerebral edema. You may also note fever, nuchal rigidity, irritability, seizures, nausea, vomiting, photophobia, focal neurologic deficits (such as hemiparesis and hemiplegia), and cranial nerve palsies (such as ptosis). When you review the history, you may find exposure to a virus that commonly causes encephalitis in the United States — arboviruses, mumps, measles, or herpes simplex, for example.

Epidural hemorrhage (acute). In this disorder, an immediate, brief loss of consciousness followed by a rapid, steady decline in LOC occur along with a progressively severe headache. In 30% to 40% of patients, the brief decline in LOC is followed by a lucid interval. These symptoms are often accompanied by nausea and vomiting, unilateral seizures, contralateral hemiparesis, hemiplegia, high fever, ipsilateral pupil dilation, and signs of increasing ICP. The patient will probably have a history of head trauma within the past 24 hours.

Heatstroke. As body temperature increases, consciousness gradually diminishes from lethargy to coma. Early signs and symptoms include malaise, tachycardia, tachypnea, orthostatic hypotension, muscle cramps, and syncope. The patient may be irritable, anxious, and dizzy, and he may report a severe headache. His skin will be hot, flushed, and diaphoretic. Later, when his core temperature exceeds 105° F (40.6° C), his skin becomes hot, flushed, and anhidrotic. Pulse and respiratory rates increase markedly, while blood pressure drops precipitously. Other findings may include vomiting, diarrhea, dilated pupils, and Cheyne-Stokes respirations. The patient will have a history of prolonged exposure to extreme heat and humidity with inadequate fluid intake.

Hepatic encephalopathy. Changes in mental status occur gradually in this disorder, with symptoms developing in four stages. In the prodromal stage, slight personality changes, disorientation, forgetfulness, slurred speech, and slight tremor occur. In the impending stage, tremor progresses to asterixis — the hallmark of hepatic encephalopathy — and lethargy, aberrant behavior, and apraxia develop. In the stuporous stage, stupor is accompanied by hyperventilation; when aroused, the patient is noisy and abusive. In the comatose stage, you may note decerebrate posture, hyperactive reflexes, positive Babinski's reflex, and fetor hepaticus. The patient may have a history of cirrhosis, liver dysfunction, sepsis, or infection. He may have recently received a sedative or general anesthetic.

Hyperglycemic hyperosmolar nonketotic coma. Cytotoxic cerebral edema causes the patient's LOC to decrease rapidly from lethargy to coma. Early findings include polyuria, polydipsia, weakness, and anorexia. Later findings include orthostatic hypotension, poor skin turgor, dry skin and mucous membranes, Kussmaul's respirations, oliguria, abdominal pain, and a rapid, thready pulse. The history will reveal Type II diabetes mellitus, possibly accompanied by an infection or other illness, and obesity.

Hypertensive encephalopathy. Vasogenic cerebral edema causes consciousness to progressively decrease from confusion and obtundation to stupor and, ultimately, coma. Besides markedly elevated blood pressure, the patient may experience severe headache, vomiting, seizures, visual disturbances, transient paralysis, and eventually Cheyne-Stokes respirations. He may not be complying with his antihypertensive regimen. Or the patient's history may include a recent hypertensive crisis, acute glomerulonephritis, or pregnancy-induced hypertension.

Hypothermia (severe). When a patient's core body temperature drops below 89.6° F (32° C), his LOC decreases rapidly from lethargy to coma. Deep tendon reflexes disappear, and ventricular fibrillation occurs. Early signs include irritability, weakness, drowsiness, lethargy, confusion, impaired coordination, ataxia, muscle stiffness, and hyperactive deep tendon reflexes. You

may also note diuresis, bradypnea, hypotension, shivering, and cold, pale skin. Later, muscle rigidity and decreased reflexes may appear, along with peripheral cyanosis, dysrhythmias, severe hypotension, decreased respiratory rate, and oliguria.

Increasing ICP. In this disorder, consciousness may diminish gradually or suddenly. Early signs include elevated blood pressure, tachycardia, altered mentation, headache, and projectile vomiting. Bradycardia occurs as a late sign of this condition, along with tachypnea or apneustic respirations and widening pulse pressure. Associated signs and symptoms include seizures and pupillary changes. Cheyne-Stokes respirations indicate deteriorating brain function. A systemic infection, head trauma, brain tumor, or underlying metabolic or cardiac disease may be part of the patient's medical history.

Intracerebral hemorrhage (acute). A rapid, steady loss of consciousness commonly progresses to coma over several hours and is accompanied by severe, generalized headache that may start suddenly or gradually. Hypertension and occasionally nuchal rigidity and vomiting may also occur. Depending on the size and location of the hemorrhage, other signs and symptoms may include hemiplegia, hemiparesis, abnormal pupil size and response, aphasia, dizziness, nausea, seizures, decreased sensations, homonymous hemianopia, urinary incontinence, visual field defects, dysphagia, dysarthria, blindness, irregular respirations, positive Babinski's reflex, and decorticate or decerebrate posture. The patient's history may include a cerebral aneurysm, congenital vascular defects, hemorrhagic disorders, hypertension, cardiovascular disease, head trauma, cocaine or stimulant abuse, blood dyscrasias, or use of anticoagulants.

Lead poisoning (chronic). Changes in LOC from cytotoxic cerebral edema progress from intermittent stupor and lucid periods to coma in the acute stage of poisoning. These changes follow anorexia, apathy, lethargy, malaise, anemia, behavior disturbances, clumsiness, developmental deterioration, persistent and forceful vomiting, seizures, and ataxia. You may note peripheral neuropathies and lead lines along the gums in an adult. The history may include ingestion of paint containing lead or illegally produced whiskey containing lead, or occupational exposure to lead.

Meningitis. With this disorder, the patient will be confused and irritable. In severe meningitis, stupor and coma may also occur, along with a sudden, severe, constant, generalized headache that worsens with movement. You may also observe nuchal rigidity and possibly fever. Associated signs include chills, positive Kernig's and Brudzinski's signs, hyperreflexia and, in some cases, opisthotonos. As ICP increases, vomiting and, occasionally, papilledema develop. Other features may include seizures, ocular palsies, facial weakness, and hearing loss. The patient's history may reveal systemic or sinus infection, dental work, or exposure to bacteria or viruses that commonly cause meningitis, such as *Haemophilus influenzae, Streptococcus pneumoniae, Neisseria meningitidis,* enteroviruses, measles, and mumps.

Myxedema coma. The alterations in LOC resulting from cytotoxic cerebral edema vary from extreme lethargy, hypersomnolence, and impaired consciousness to deep coma. Associated findings include severe hypothermia, hypoventilation, hypotension, bradycardia, hypoactive reflexes, periorbital and peripheral edema, and seizures. The patient may be elderly, have a history of prolonged hypothyroidism, and have been exposed to the cold, experienced trauma, contracted an infection, or used central nervous system depressants.

Pontine hemorrhage. The patient's LOC suddenly plummets into coma immediately after hemorrhage. Within minutes, death may occur. The patient shows accompanying signs of total paralysis, absence of doll's eye sign, a positive Babinski's reflex, and small, nonreactive pupils. The patient's history will probably include head trauma or unmanaged hypertension.

Reye's syndrome. In this disorder, which follows viral disease in a child, lethargy, stupor, and coma replace hyperexcitability. The patient may experience severe and repetitive vomiting, fever, and seizures over a period of a few days. His history will probably include recent influenza (particularly type B) or chicken pox, possibly accompanied by aspirin ingestion.

Shock. Confusion, lethargy, and restlessness progressing to stupor and coma result from the ischemic cerebral edema of shock. Associated findings include anxiety, hypotension, tachycardia, weak pulse with narrowing pulse pressure, dyspnea, oliguria, and cool, clammy skin. Chest pain or dysrhythmias and signs of congestive heart failure (such as dyspnea, cough, edema, distended neck veins, and weight gain) may also occur with cardiogenic shock. Fever and chills may accompany septic shock. The patient's history may indicate the cause of shock, such as exposure to an allergen (anaphylactic shock), internal or external hemorrhage (hypovolemic shock), recent myocardial infarction (cardiogenic shock), severe systemic infection (septic shock), or spinal cord injury (neurogenic shock).

Subarachnoid hemorrhage. In this disorder, an altered LOC may progress rapidly to coma. Accompanying signs and symptoms may include sudden, violent headache; nuchal rigidity; nausea; vomiting; seizures; dizziness; hypertension; and ipsilateral pupil dilation. The patient will also have positive Kernig's and Brudzinski's signs, photophobia, blurred vision, and possibly fever. Focal signs and symptoms, such as hemiparesis, hemiplegia, sensory or vision disturbances, and aphasia, may occur, as may other signs of elevated ICP. The patient may have a history of congenital vascular defects (such as arteriovenous malformation), underlying cardiovascular disease, cocaine use, smoking, excessive stress, or excessive caffeine intake.

Subdural hematoma (acute). Typically this disorder follows recent head trauma. The patient's LOC progressively decreases from agitation and confusion to somnolence and coma. This is accompanied by a severe, localized headache. Other signs and symptoms, which may occur later, include indications of increased ICP, ipsilateral pupillary dilation progressing to fixation, coma, and focal neurologic deficits,

such as hemiparesis. The patient's history may include head trauma within 3 days of the onset of symptoms with acute subdural hematoma, within 3 weeks of onset with subacute hematoma, and over 3 weeks with chronic hematoma. About half of the patients have no history of head trauma.

Other causes
Certain causes of decreased LOC may not require immediate intervention.

Disorders. An altered LOC can occur in any condition affecting the patient's brain function. These include acute febrile illness in children, brain tumor, cerebrovascular accident, chronic subdural hematoma, dementia, hydrocephalus, hypercapnia with pulmonary disease, hyperventilation syndrome, hypokalemia, hyponatremia, low perfusion states, migraine headache, nutritional deficiencies, poisoning, seizures, status epilepticus, and transient ischemic attack.

Drugs. Sedation and other degrees of decreased LOC can result from central nervous system depressants, such as barbiturates, antihistamines, and anticholinergics. Use of alcohol and street drugs causes varying degrees of sedation, irritability, impaired judgment, and incoordination; intoxication commonly leads to stupor and coma.

Oliguria

Urine output of less than 400 ml/24 hours is referred to as oliguria. This sign can develop gradually as renal tissue destruction impairs

Stress triggers oliguria

Whenever the body undergoes stress, the endocrine and autonomic nervous systems boost their secretion of most hormones. As the level of antidiuretic hormone rises, the kidneys conserve water. Thus, a person under stress experiences water retention and oliguria.

Any type of stress can induce this compensatory response—particularly when it's accompanied by infection and hypovolemia.

kidney function (intrarenal). Or oliguria can occur abruptly when low renal blood perfusion decreases the kidneys' ability to produce urine (prerenal) or when an obstruction prevents urine from being eliminated (postrenal). (For more information on the pathophysiology of these three types of oliguria, see *How oliguria develops*. Also, see *Stress triggers oliguria*.)

Usually, oliguria resulting from a prerenal or postrenal cause can be quickly reversed. If left untreated, however, such oliguria may lead to intrarenal damage. When oliguria results from an intrarenal cause, it's usually more persistent and may be irreversible.

History questions
Explore the patient's problem by asking appropriate questions from this section. (For more information, see *Case in point: A blocked catheter mimics acute renal failure*, page 128.)

• Ask the patient to describe his usual daily voiding pattern, including how often and how much he urinates. Does he have difficulty starting or maintaining urination? Also ask him to estimate how much fluid he drinks daily.

• When did he first notice a change in this pattern? Did it develop suddenly or gradually? Has he recently been drinking more or less fluid than usual? Does he feel any pain or burning on urination? Has he noticed any change in the color, odor, or consistency of his urine? If so, ask him to describe the changes.

• Has the patient had recent episodes of diarrhea or vomiting? Is he experiencing other associated symptoms—especially fatigue, nausea, loss of appetite, thirst, dyspnea, chest pain, or weight gain?

• Does the patient have any pain, particularly a headache or flank, abdominal, or pelvic pain? Have him describe the pain. Did it start at the same time as the oliguria? Earlier? Later?

• Is the patient pregnant? If so, has she had a sudden weight gain, dizziness, blurred vision, diplopia, irritability, or a severe frontal headache? Has she had a similar episode during a previous pregnancy?

• Does the patient have a condition that can cause shock, such as sepsis, hypovolemia, severe trauma, myocardial infarction, or spinal cord injury? What about exposure to an allergen?

• Has the patient been exposed to nephrotoxic agents—heavy metals, industrial solvents, pesticides, or fungicides?

• Has the patient had abdominal, pelvic, renal, or urinary tract surgery? Has he recently undergone any diagnostic tests that use contrast media or received methoxyflurane as an anesthetic for surgery? These drugs may also cause nephrotoxicity?

• Is the patient taking, or has he recently taken, any other drugs that may cause nephrotoxicity? Such drugs include aminoglycosides,

PATHOPHYSIOLOGY

How oliguria develops

This flowchart shows you the pathophysiology of the three types of oliguria.

PRERENAL CAUSES	**INTRARENAL CAUSES**	**POSTRENAL CAUSES**
• Adhesions	• Acute glomerulonephritis	• Adhesions
• Bilateral renal artery occlusion	• Acute tubular necrosis	• Benign prostatic hypertrophy
• Bilateral renal vein occlusion	• Pregnancy-induced hypertension	• Bladder dysfunction
• Low perfusion states	• Nephrotoxic agents	• Calculi
• Shock	• Renal failure	• Strictures
	• Renal tumors	• Tumors
		• Catheter obstruction

Prerenal pathway:

Hypoperfusion

↓

Decreased glomerular filtration rate

↓

Increased proximal tubular reabsorption of sodium and water

↓

Increased secretion of aldosterone and antidiuretic hormone

↓

Increased distal tubular reabsorption of sodium and water

Intrarenal pathway:

Damage to renal tubules

↓ ↓

Increased renal vasoconstriction | Intratubular obstruction

↓ | ↓

Cellular edema | Increased intratubular pressure

↓ | ↓

Decreased glomerular capillary permeability | Leakage of tubular fluid into interstitium

↓

Decreased glomerular filtration rate

↓

Tubular dysfunction

Postrenal pathway:

Obstruction of urine flow

↓

Backup of urine

↓

Compression of renal tubules

OLIGURIA

EMERGENCY INTERVENTION

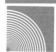

Case in point: A blocked catheter mimics acute renal failure

By failing to make a rapid, systematic assessment of your patient, you can misread symptoms as life-threatening when in fact they're not. That's just what happened to Janice Robinson, a nurse caring for Fred Wise, age 64.

Mr. Wise's condition was just beginning to stabilize after a recent myocardial infarction complicated by cardiogenic shock. Janice was monitoring his hourly urine output to detect oliguria—a sign that could indicate acute renal failure.

Failure to assess

Over a 7-hour period, Mr. Wise's urine output totaled only 120 ml, even though his intake was 600 ml. Janice suspected that low renal perfusion resulting from cardiogenic shock was the cause of Mr. Wise's acute renal failure.

She immediately documented her findings and called the doctor without making any further assessment of the patient.

When the doctor examined Mr. Wise, he found that the oliguria wasn't caused by acute renal failure but by a blocked indwelling urinary catheter. After being irrigated, the catheter drained 750 ml.

Evaluating the care

With a more thorough assessment, Janice probably would have identified Mr. Wise's problem herself. Here's the procedure you should follow in this situation.

First, ask the patient if he's having any pain. Usually, a distended bladder will cause pelvic discomfort or severe pain if the distention causes bladder spasms. Next, examine the color of the urine. If it's clear yellow or light amber, the problem probably isn't impaired renal function. You could also test the specific gravity. If it falls between 1.005 and 1.020, renal function is probably adequate.

With any patient who has an indwelling catheter, always rule out a mechanical cause for oliguria by palpating and percussing the bladder for distention. Also, irrigate the catheter to remove any obstruction that could be preventing drainage.

Then, assess the patient's neurologic status. If he has renal failure, he'll probably show signs of impaired neurologic function.

In short, you should always perform a rapid but complete nursing assessment before deciding whether or not a true emergency exists.

---

amphotericin B, and sulfonamides. What about drugs that may cause urinary tract calculi or obstructive uropathy, such as acetazolamide, methysergide, or vitamin D?

Physical examination

Base your assessment of the patient on the health history information you've collected.

Inspection. Assess the patient's overall appearance, noting the amount of edema as a baseline. Inspect for any signs of dehydration, such as decreased skin turgor. To check for neurologic toxicity, observe the patient's level of consciousness (LOC).

Inspect the rate and depth of his respirations. Note any breathing difficulty and any abnormal respiratory patterns. Next, observe his flank for edema, erythema, or signs of renal trauma, such as Cullen's or Turner's sign.

Check the patient's urine for abnormal color, odor, or sediment. Then test it for glucose, protein, blood, and specific gravity.

Palpation. Note the rate, rhythm, and intensity of the peripheral pulses. Then palpate both kidneys for tenderness and enlargement. To rule out urine retention, palpate the bladder; to rule out hepatomegaly, palpate the liver.

Percussion. Check for pain or tenderness by percussing over the costovertebral angle. Percuss over the bladder for fullness or distention.

Auscultation. Monitor the patient's blood pressure and note any changes in his pulse pressure. Auscultate the heart and lungs for abnormal sounds and the periumbilical area for renal artery bruits.

Life-threatening causes

Your assessment may lead you to suspect one or more of the following.

Acute tubular necrosis. An early sign of acute tubular necrosis (ATN), oliguria may occur abruptly, as in ischemia or infarction, or gradually, as in nephrotoxicity. Signs of neurologic toxicity (confusion and decreasing LOC), hyperkalemia (muscle weakness and cardiac dysrhythmias), and uremia (anorexia, confusion, lethargy, twitching, seizures, pruritus, and Kussmaul's respirations) soon follow. The patient's history may reveal a condition that can cause ATN, such as circulatory collapse, severe hypotension, trauma, hemorrhage, shock, renal artery or vein occlusion, or transfusion reaction. The patient may have been exposed to such

nephrotoxins as antibiotics, contrast media, pesticides, fungicides, heavy metals, or industrial solvents.

Glomerulonephritis (acute). Oliguria or anuria occurs rarely in this disorder and usually indicates a poor prognosis. Common signs include hematuria, mild fever, fatigue, generalized edema and possibly anasarca, elevated blood pressure, headache, nausea, vomiting, and flank and abdominal pain. Hypervolemia causes mild to moderate hypertension and circulatory and pulmonary congestion, resulting in dyspnea, orthopnea, crackles, and a productive cough. The patient's history usually includes pharyngitis 1 to 3 weeks before symptoms begin. But in some cases, the patient's history won't reveal an obvious precipitating cause.

Pregnancy-induced hypertension. In severe preeclampsia, oliguria may be accompanied by elevated blood pressure, dizziness, diplopia, blurred vision, epigastric pain, nausea and vomiting, irritability, and a severe frontal headache. Typically, the oliguria follows generalized edema and sudden weight gain of more than 3 pounds per week during the second trimester or more than 1 pound per week during the third trimester. If preeclampsia progresses to eclampsia, the patient has seizures and may slip into coma. Her history may include excessive weight gain or peripheral edema during the pregnancy or a similar episode in a previous pregnancy.

Shock. Oliguria resulting from decreased perfusion to the kidneys occurs in this condition. You may also note anxiety, hypotension, tachycardia, a weak pulse with narrowing pulse pressure, dyspnea, a decreased LOC, and cool, clammy skin. Chest pain or dysrhythmias and signs of congestive heart failure—dyspnea, cough, edema, distended neck veins, and weight gain—may also occur with cardiogenic shock. Fever and chills may accompany septic shock. The patient's history may explain the cause of the shock: exposure to an allergen (anaphylactic shock), internal or external hemorrhage (hypovolemic shock), recent myocardial infarction (cardiogenic shock), severe systemic infection (septic shock), or spinal cord injury (neurogenic shock).

Other causes
Certain causes of oliguria may not signal the need for immediate intervention.

Diagnostic studies. A patient undergoing a radiographic study that uses contrast media may develop nephrotoxicity and oliguria.

Disorders. Oliguria may accompany adhesions, benign prostatic hypertrophy, bladder dysfunction, calculi, congenital hydronephrosis, dehydration, hemolytic uremic syndrome, hepatorenal syndrome, chronic renal failure, respiratory distress syndrome, ureteral or urethral stricture, or urinary tract, abdominal, or pelvic tumors.

Drugs. Oliguria may result from drugs that cause decreased renal perfusion (diuretics), nephrotoxicity (most notably, aminoglycosides and chemotherapeutic agents such as cisplatin and methotrexate), urine retention (adrenergic and anticholinergic agents), or urinary obstruction associated with urinary crystals (sulfonamides).

Palpitations

Defined as a person's conscious awareness of his own heartbeat, palpitations are usually felt over the precordium or in the throat or neck. The patient may describe his heart as pounding, jumping, turning, fluttering, or flopping, or as missing or skipping beats. Palpitations may be regular or irregular, fast or slow, paroxysmal or sustained.

History questions
Explore the patient's problem by asking appropriate questions from this section.
• What was the patient doing when the palpitations started? How long did they last? Has he experienced similar episodes before? Are the symptoms and the precipitating event similar?
• Is the patient having any chest pain, dizziness, or weakness along with the palpitations? Is he experiencing other symptoms, such as spasms in the feet and hands, muscle cramps, or numbness and tingling of the fingertips, feet, or mouth? Ask too about anorexia, weakness, fatigue, exertional dyspnea, muscle tremor, and confusion. If the patient is a woman, has she noticed decreased or absent menses?
• Has the patient recently undergone multiple blood transfusions or an infusion of phosphate?
• Does the patient have a history of thyroid disease, hypoparathyroidism, pseudohypoparathyroidism, calcium or vitamin D deficiency, malabsorption syndrome, acute pancreatitis, bone malignancy, or renal disease? How about cardiovascular or pulmonary disorders that may

produce dysrhythmias? Hypertension or hypoglycemia?

• Ask about his drug history. Has he recently started digitalis therapy? Is he taking an over-the-counter drug containing caffeine or a sympathomimetic, such as a cough, cold, or allergy preparation? Also, ask about tobacco and alcohol consumption.

Physical examination

Base your assessment of the patient on the health history information you've collected.

Inspection. Check the patient's skin for pallor or diaphoresis, then look for exophthalmos. As you observe his respirations, note their rate and depth. Does he have any difficulty breathing? Is his respiratory pattern normal?

Assess the patient's level of consciousness, noting any confusion, anxiety, nervousness, or irrational behavior. Also, inspect his fingertips for capillary nail bed pulsations.

Palpation. Gently palpate the neck for thyroid enlargement. Keep in mind that excessive thyroid manipulation in the hyperthyroid patient can precipitate thyrotoxicosis. Then, palpate the patient's muscles for weakness or twitching. Check his peripheral pulses, noting rate, rhythm, and intensity.

Percussion. Assess the patient's reflexes. Do you detect any hyperreflexia? Check for a positive Chvostek's or Trousseau's sign.

Auscultation. Listen over the heart for gallops and murmurs and over the lungs for abnormal breath sounds. Be sure to monitor the patient's blood pressure and pulse pressure.

Life-threatening causes

Your assessment may lead you to suspect one or more of the following.

Cardiac dysrhythmias. Paroxysmal or sustained palpitations may occur with dizziness, weakness, and fatigue. Other signs and symptoms may include decreased blood pressure, chest pain, confusion, pallor, diaphoresis, and an irregular, rapid, or slow pulse rate. The patient may be using drugs that can cause cardiac dysrhythmias — for instance, digitalis glycosides, sympathomimetics, ganglionic blockers, anticholinergics, or methylxanthines.

Hypocalcemic tetany. A decreased serum calcium level causes the neuromuscular irritability of this condition, which leads to palpitations and other signs and symptoms. These include carpopedal spasm; muscle weakness, twitching, and cramping; laryngospasm; stridor; tonic clonic seizures (mainly in children); paresthesia of the fingers, toes, and circumoral area; hyperreflexia; chorea; fatigue; and positive Chvostek's and Trousseau's signs. You may also observe signs and symptoms of the underlying disorder. The patient's history may include recent GI or thyroid surgery, vitamin D deficiency, acute pancreatitis, or metastatic bone cancer. The patient may have hypoparathyroidism and not comply with his medical regimen. Or he may have an increased serum phosphate concentration caused by either uremia, leukemia chemotherapy, or phosphate infusion.

Thyrotoxicosis (thyroid storm). A characteristic symptom of this disorder, sustained palpitations occur along with a sudden elevation of systolic pressure, widened pulse pressure, tachycardia, bounding pulse, pulsations in the capillary nail beds, and diarrhea that often results in dehydration. Other findings will include exophthalmos, an enlarged thyroid gland, fever over 100° F (37.7° C), and warm, moist skin. The patient may appear nervous and emotionally unstable, displaying occasional outbursts or even psychotic behavior. You may also note heat intolerance, exertional dyspnea, and in women, a history of decreased or absent menses. In a person with latent hyperthyroidism, the history may include excessive dietary intake of iodine and repeated episodes of symptoms following stressful conditions, such as surgery, infections, pregnancy, or diabetic ketoacidosis.

Other causes
Certain causes of palpitations may not signal the need for immediate intervention.

Disorders. Palpitations can occur in an acute anxiety attack, anemia, aortic insufficiency, hypertension, hypoglycemia, mitral prolapse, mitral stenosis, mitral regurgitation, or pheochromocytoma. Transient palpitations can accompany emotional stress — fright, anger, or anxiety — or physical stress, such as exercise or fever.

Drugs. Palpitations may be induced by drugs that precipitate cardiac dysrhythmias or increase cardiac output, such as digitalis glycosides, sympathomimetics, ganglionic blockers, and atropine. Palpitations can also result from stimulants, including tobacco, caffeine, cocaine, methamphetamines, and methylxanthines.

Prosthetic device. Nonpathologic palpitations may be reported by a patient with a newly implanted prosthetic valve because its clicking sound heightens the patient's awareness of his heartbeat.

Posturing changes

Certain distinct changes in the patient's posturing reflect brain stem ischemia or damage resulting from trauma or increasing intracranial pressure (ICP). These changes occur in a stuporous or comatose patient and are accompanied by signs of neurologic deterioration and the underlying disorder.

Depending on the level of brain or brain stem involvement, posturing changes can progress from decorticate rigidity (abnormal flexor response) to decerebrate rigidity (abnormal extensor reflex) to flaccidity. (See *Comparing abnormal postures.*) Because children under age 2 have immature nervous systems, they may not display decerebrate posture. But they may exhibit opisthotonos. In fact, opisthotonos, usually a terminal sign, is more common in infants and young children than in adults.

A noxious stimulus may trigger posturing changes. The intensity of the stimulus needed to elicit the response, the duration of the posture, and the frequency of episodes vary with the severity of cerebral injury. Usually, the longer the posturing, the greater the damage.

In some cases, decerebrate posture will affect one side of the body, while decorticate posture affects the other. The two postures may also alternate as the patient's neurologic status fluctuates. Although a serious sign, decorticate posture

Comparing abnormal postures

Any of these three postures may indicate severe neurologic damage.

DECORTICATE POSTURE

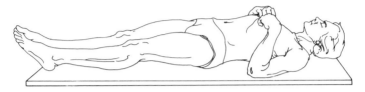

When lesions of the cerebral hemispheres or internal capsule interrupt the corti-cospinal pathways, the patient assumes the decorticate posture. His arms are adducted and flexed, his wrists and fingers are flexed on the chest, and his legs are stiffly extended and internally rotated with plantar flexion of the feet.

DECEREBRATE POSTURE

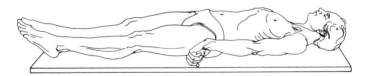

Rostral-to-caudal deterioration with midbrain or pons damage leads to decere-brate posture. Here the patient's arms are adducted and extended, with his wrists pronated and fingers flexed. The legs are stiffly extended with plantar flex-ion of the feet.

OPISTHOTONOS

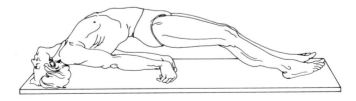

In opisthotonos, the patient's back is acutely arched, his head is bent back on his neck, his heels are bent back on his legs, and his hands and arms are flexed rigidly at the joints. Most commonly seen in children under age 2, this posture may be interpreted as a severe case of decerebrate posture.

carries a more favorable prognosis than decerebrate posture. If damage extends into the brain stem, however, decorticate posture may progress to decerebrate posture.

Primary damage to the brain stem, such as that occurring with infarction or hemorrhage, is fatal. So the patient may die before exhibiting all the posturing changes that signal each stage of deterioration.

History questions

Explore the patient's problem by asking appropriate questions from this section. Because the patient will be comatose, you'll have to obtain information from a family member, someone who brought him to the hospital, or the hospital record.

• When did the patient's level of consciousness begin deteriorating? Did it happen slowly or abruptly? Did a specific event precede the loss of consciousness? For instance, did the patient suffer a head injury?

• Did the patient complain of other symptoms before he lost consciousness? Perhaps nausea, vertigo, or headache?

• Has the patient been exposed to poisonous substances? Does he have a history of drug or alcohol abuse?

• Does he have a history of endocrine, hepatic, renal, neurologic, or cardiovascular disease? How about cancer, anoxia, or electrolyte or acid-base imbalances?

Physical examination

Base your assessment of the patient on the health history information you've collected.

Inspection. Check if the size of the patient's pupils is the same. Do they react to light? Perform the doll's eye maneuver, checking for eye movement and dysconjugate gaze.

Observe his respirations, noting their rate and depth. Does he have difficulty breathing? Do you see an abnormal respiratory pattern — Cheyne-Stokes or apneustic respirations, central neurogenic hyperventilation, ataxic respirations, or apnea, for instance?

Palpation. Check the rate, rhythm, and intensity of peripheral pulses.

Percussion. Stimulate the patient and note the degree and duration of posturing. Check his deep tendon reflexes, comparing responses bilaterally. Note any abnormal responses.

Auscultation. Monitor the patient's blood pressure and pulse pressure.

Life-threatening cause

Your assessment may lead you to suspect this disorder.

Increased ICP. Decorticate posture occurs when ICP increases enough to compress the midbrain. Usually, this condition is accompanied by pupils that are in the midposition and fixed, as well as absent doll's eye sign, dysconjugate gaze, Cheyne-Stokes respirations or central neurogenic hyperventilation, and wide variations in body temperature. The patient may also have diabetes insipidus.

Decerebrate posture occurs when the increased pressure affects the pons. Usually, this is accompanied by pupils that are small and fixed, central neurogenic hyperventilation or apneustic respirations, elevated temperature, and an erratic pulse. You may also note absent doll's eye sign and a dysconjugate gaze.

Progressive neurologic deterioration of the medulla causes ataxic respirations, followed by apnea, flaccidity, and an absent pulse.

Deterioration may occur gradually or suddenly, depending on the cause of the increasing ICP. Early signs may include elevated blood pressure, bradycardia, widened pulse pressure, altered mentation, progressive loss of consciousness, persistent headache, projectile vomiting, and seizures. You may also note signs and symptoms of the underlying disorder. The patient's history may include a systemic or brain infection, head trauma, brain tumor, or underlying metabolic or cardiovascular disease.

Other causes

In rare cases, some neurologic tests can cause increased ICP, brain stem compression, and, eventually, posturing changes. Such procedures include lumbar puncture, cisternography, and pneumoencephalography.

Pulse, absent or weak

An absent or weak pulse may be generalized, or it may affect only one limb. When generalized, this sign usually indicates low cardiac output. A localized loss or weakness of a usually strong pulse may indicate arterial occlusion. (See *Managing a weak or absent pulse*, pages 136 and 137.)

Sometimes, a normal pulse may be misinterpreted as absent or weak. That's because palpation can temporarily diminish or obliterate a superficial pulse, such as the posterior tibial or the dorsal pedal. So remember, bilateral weakness or absence of these pulses isn't necessarily abnormal.

To avoid misinterpretation when assessing infants and small children, evaluate arterial circulation to the limbs by palpating the brachial, popliteal, or femoral pulse. In these patients, the radial, dorsal pedal, and posterior tibial pulses aren't easy to palpate. If you use them, you may mistake a hard-to-palpate pulse for an absent or weak one.

History questions

Explore the patient's problem by asking appropriate questions from this section. If emergency treatment is needed, ask questions as you intervene.
• Does the patient have accompanying signs and symptoms, such as dyspnea, light-headedness, fatigue, anxiety, a feeling of impending doom, itching, weakness, palpitations, dizziness, nausea, vomiting, diarrhea, chills, or cool, clammy skin? Does he have a cough? If so, is it productive?
• Is the patient in pain? If so, ask him to describe it. Where is it? Did it start suddenly or gradually? Does it radiate? Does it get better or worse with activity?
• Has the patient recently experienced trauma or undergone surgery? Has he had a systemic infection?
• Does he have a history of cardiovascular, pulmonary, or GI disease? If he has allergies, has he been exposed to allergens?
• What medications is he taking?

Physical examination

Base your assessment of the patient on the health history information you've collected.

Inspection. While examining his skin, note diaphoresis, lines of frank demarcation, mottling, pallor, or flushing. Also, check the skin temperature. If an arm or leg is cool and pale, elevate it slightly and

(Text continues on page 138.)

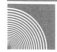

Managing a weak or absent pulse

Sometimes, when a patient's pulse is weak or absent, you may need to intervene immediately. Exactly how you assess and intervene will depend on whether the problem pulse is generalized or localized and on the associated signs and symptoms. To help you establish priorities for managing this emergency successfully, use this flowchart.

GENERALIZED WEAK OR ABSENT PULSE

Patient is confused and restless; has hypotension and cool, pale, clammy skin.

• History of trauma • Excessive thirst • Flat neck veins • Narrowed pulse pressure	• History of myocardial infarction (MI) or congestive heart failure • Distended neck veins • Ventricular gallop • Crackles • Narrowed pulse pressure	• History of recent cardiac surgery or catheterization, chest trauma, pericardial effusion, or anticoagulant therapy • Distended neck veins • Pulsus paradoxus • Muffled heart sounds	• History of MI or chronic heart or lung disease • Irregular heart rate • Severe tachycardia or bradycardia • Palpitations
▽ Suspect hypovolemic shock.	▽ Suspect cardiogenic shock.	▽ Suspect cardiac tamponade.	▽ Suspect dysrhythmias.
▽	▽	▽	▽

Immediately inform the doctor. Administer oxygen by nasal cannula and insert an I.V. line for fluid infusion. Begin cardiac monitoring and check vital signs every 5 to 15 minutes. If ordered, assist with insertion of a central venous pressure line, an arterial line, or a pulmonary artery catheter. Be prepared for emergency resuscitation, if necessary.

▽ Anticipate colloid or crystalloid replacement, or both.	▽ Anticipate administering nitroprusside and dopamine simultaneously.	▽ Anticipate pericardiocentesis.	▽ Anticipate administering antiarrhythmics.

LOCALIZED WEAK OR ABSENT PULSE

Cool, mottled skin and pain in affected arm or leg → Suspect arterial occlusive disease. → Inform the doctor. Prepare for arteriography or ultrasonography. Don't elevate the affected arm or leg. Prepare for thrombolytic therapy or surgery. Start an I.V. line in an unaffected arm or leg.

Patient is confused and restless; has hypotension and cool, pale, clammy skin.

• History of trauma, congenital heart disease, or hypertension • Severe, tearing chest pain • Unequal peripheral pulses	• History of severe infection • Fever • Chills • Widened pulse pressure	• History of an insect sting, drug ingestion, or exposure to another possible allergen • Urticaria • Wheezing or stridor • Dyspnea	• History of venous stasis or deep vein thrombosis • Sharp, substernal chest pain • Dyspnea, crackles • Pleural friction rub • Hemoptysis
▽	▽	▽	▽
Suspect dissecting aortic aneurysm.	Suspect septic shock.	Suspect anaphylactic shock.	Suspect pulmonary embolism.
▽	▽	▽	▽

Immediately inform the doctor. Administer oxygen by nasal cannula and insert an I.V. line for fluid infusion. Begin cardiac monitoring and check vital signs every 5 to 15 minutes. If ordered, assist with insertion of a central venous pressure line, an arterial line, or a pulmonary artery catheter. Be prepared for emergency resuscitation, if necessary.

▽	▽	▽	▽
Anticipate preparing the patient for surgery and administering an antihypertensive or nitroprusside.	Anticipate administering antibiotics and vasopressors.	Anticipate emergency intubation or cricothyrotomy and administration of epinephrine.	Anticipate possible intubation and anticoagulant or thrombolytic therapy.

observe for cadaveric pallor in the toes or feet. Then check for prolonged (longer than 2 seconds) capillary refill time.

Observe the patient's respirations, noting their rate and depth. Does he have difficulty breathing or an abnormal breathing pattern? During the respiratory cycle, listen for stridor or hoarseness. Note any blood-tinged sputum produced from coughing.

Then, inspect the patient's neck for jugular vein distention. Assess his level of consciousness, noting restlessness, confusion, anxiety, or seizures. Be sure to measure his abdominal girth and monitor for any increase. To check for muscle weakness, hemiplegia, or focal neurologic deficits, observe his motor activity. Examine him for signs of trauma, such as bruising, erythema, and abrasions. Monitor his urine output for oliguria or anuria.

Palpation. As you palpate the peripheral pulses, note their rate, rhythm, and intensity. Palpate the abdomen for rigidity, pain, and tenderness. If you note any guarding, gently palpate the area for a mass or hepatomegaly. If you detect a palpable mass, does it pulsate?

Percussion. Carefully percuss the abdomen. Note any areas of tympany, hyperresonance, or dullness. Gently percuss the chest and back, listening for areas of dullness.

Auscultation. Listen to the patient's lungs for abnormal breath sounds. Especially note diminished sounds, rhonchi, wheezes, crackles, and pleural friction rubs.

Auscultate the heart for abnormal sounds, particularly faint or muffled heart sounds, murmurs, gallops, or pericardial friction rubs. Then,

auscultate the abdomen for aortic bruits and bowel sounds.

Monitor the patient's blood pressure and pulse pressure. Also, monitor the intensity of Korotkoff's sounds. To detect orthostatic hypotension, measure his blood pressure while he's supine and while he sits.

Life-threatening causes
Your assessment may lead you to suspect one or more of the following.

Anaphylactic shock. Generalized weak pulses develop suddenly from a dramatic fall in blood pressure and a narrowed pulse pressure. This usually follows extreme anxiety, restlessness, feelings of impending doom, intense itching (especially of the hands and feet), and a pounding headache. Symptoms usually start within seconds or minutes of exposure to an allergen; however, delayed reactions of up to 24 hours may occur. Later, anaphylactic shock may also produce flushing, cardiac dysrhythmias, tachycardia, seizures, coughing, sneezing, dyspnea, nasal congestion, stridor and hoarseness from laryngeal edema, as well as nausea, abdominal cramps, involuntary defecation, and urinary incontinence. The patient may have allergies or a family history of them. Or he may have a history of exposure to a known or common allergen. For instance, he may have been stung by a bee or taken such drugs as penicillins or sulfonamides.

Aortic aneurysm (dissecting). A weak or absent femoral or pedal pulse may be unilateral in this disorder. Associated signs and symptoms vary, depending on whether the patient has an abdominal or thoracic aneurysm. With an abdominal aneurysm, the patient may experience persistent abdominal and back pain, weakness, sweating, tachycardia, dyspnea, restlessness, and confusion. You may note mottled skin below the waist, increasing abdominal girth, abdominal rigidity, and cool, clammy skin. On auscultation, you may find a systolic bruit. And on palpation, you may detect tenderness over the area of the aneurysm and an epigastric mass that pulsates before rupturing.

With a thoracic aneurysm, the patient will feel a severe ripping or tearing pain in his chest, which radiates to the neck, shoulders, lower back, or abdomen. This may be accompanied by pallor, syncope, sweating, dyspnea, tachycardia, cyanosis, leg weakness, and a sudden onset of neurologic symptoms. Auscultation may reveal a murmur suggesting aortic regurgitation. Other findings may include weakness or transient paralysis of the legs, the diastolic murmur of aortic insufficiency, hypotension, and mottled skin below the waist. Blood pressure may be lower in the patient's legs than in his arms or may be different in each arm. He may be diaphoretic and have prolonged capillary refill time in his feet. His history will likely include smoking as well as claudication and other symptoms of cardiovascular disease.

Aortic bifurcation occlusion (acute). With this disorder, femoral, popliteal, and pedal pulses will be absent in both legs. These signs will be accompanied by sudden ischemic pain, sensory and motor deficits distal to the obstruction, and cadaveric pallor of the toes and feet even when they're elevated slightly. The patient may also complain of pain in the abdomen, lumbosacral area, or perineum. He'll probably have a history of smoking and cardiovascular disease.

Arterial limb occlusion (acute). Pulses distal to the obstruction are weak and eventually disappear. A line of color and temperature demarcation develops at the level of obstruction. With a more ischemic limb, the patient will feel pain at rest, and you'll note a cadaveric pallor when the limb is elevated even slightly. Varying degrees of limb paralysis can also develop along with intense intermittent claudication. The patient's history may include recent surgery, trauma, or cardiovascular disease.

Cardiac dysrhythmias. With this disorder, you'll note generalized weak pulses and cool, clammy skin. Other signs and symptoms reflect the type and severity of the dysrhythmia. These may include hypotension, chest pain, dizziness, and a decreased level of consciousness. Low blood pressure may alternate with normal readings and may be accompanied by light-headedness, weakness, fatigue, and palpitations. Auscultation typically reveals a pulse rate greater than 100 beats/minute or less than 60 beats/minute, or an irregular rhythm. The patient's history may reveal previous cardiac disease.

Cardiac tamponade. As the pericardium fills with blood or fluid, weak and rapid peripheral pulses may be accompanied by these classic findings: pulsus paradoxus, jugular vein distention, hypotension, narrowed pulse pressure, and muffled heart sounds. However, some hypovolemic patients may not have jugular vein distention, and if the patient is sitting upright, his heart sounds may not be muffled. The patient may appear anxious, restless, and cyanotic. He may also have chest pain, clammy skin, dyspnea, and tachypnea. You may note pericardial friction rubs and hepatomegaly. The health history may include recent chest trauma, pericarditis, myocardial infarction, fever, malaise, chronic tamponade, or treatment with anticoagulants.

Cardiogenic shock. Depending on the degree of vascular collapse, peripheral pulses may be absent and central pulses weak. You may also see a decrease in systolic pressure to less than 80 mm Hg or 30 mm Hg less than the patient's baseline. Other signs and symptoms include a narrowed pulse pressure, diminished Korotkoff's sounds, peripheral cyanosis, restlessness, anxiety that can progress to disorientation and confusion, and pale, cool, clammy skin. You may also detect anginal pain, dyspnea, jugular vein distention, and oliguria. Auscultation may reveal tachypnea, tachycardia, faint heart sounds, ventricular gallop, and possibly a systolic murmur. The patient's history may include disorders that cause left ventricular dysfunction.

Hypovolemic shock. Depending on the severity of the hypovolemia, peripheral pulses become weak, then uniformly absent. As shock progresses, the remaining pulses become thready and more rapid. Systolic pressure falls to less than 80 mm Hg or 30 mm Hg less than the patient's baseline. This drop is accompanied by orthostatic pressure changes, diminished Korotkoff's sounds, narrowed pulse pressure, and tachypnea and tachycardia, which increase as blood volume de-

creases. Other symptoms include angina (in patients with coronary artery disease), light-headedness, irritability, diaphoresis, extreme thirst, hypothermia, decreased capillary refill, confusion, disorientation, restlessness, and anxiety. Decreased renal perfusion causes oliguria and peripheral vasoconstriction, leading to cyanosis of the limbs and pale, cool, clammy skin. The patient's history may include trauma, GI disorders, internal bleeding, burns, or extended periods of perspiration, diarrhea, or vomiting.

Neurogenic shock. Uniformly weak pulses accompanying hypotension and bradycardia are the cardinal signs of neurogenic shock, although in most cases systolic pressure doesn't fall below 100 mm Hg. Vasodilation occurring in neurogenic shock causes the relative hypovolemia that produces the symptoms. Vasodilation also causes the skin to remain warm, dry, and flushed. The patient's history will reveal a condition that can cause neurogenic shock, such as spinal cord injury.

Pulmonary embolism. A generalized weak, rapid pulse may accompany the sudden dyspnea that's the hallmark of this disorder. You may also find sudden angina-like or pleuritic pain aggravated by deep breathing and thoracic movement. Accompanying signs and symptoms include hypotension, apprehension, restlessness, syncope, and diaphoresis. Other findings are anxiety, tachypnea, decreased breath sounds, crackles, a nonproductive cough or one that produces blood-tinged sputum, a low-grade fever, pleural friction rubs, diffuse wheezing, dullness on percussion, signs of cerebral ischemia (transient unconsciousness, coma, seizures) and, particularly in the elderly, hemiplegia and other focal neurologic deficits. Central cyanosis occurs when a large embolus causes significant obstruction of the pulmonary circulation. The patient's history may include thrombophlebitis of the deep systemic veins, varicose veins, hip or leg fractures, acute myocardial infarction, congestive heart failure, cardiogenic shock, congestive cardiomyopathies, chronic atrial fibrillation, pregnancy, or use of oral contraceptives.

Septic shock. Depending on the degree of vascular collapse, pulses become weak and then may become uniformly absent. Shock is heralded by chills, sudden fever, and possibly nausea, vomiting, and diarrhea. Typically, the skin is flushed, warm, and dry. Tachycardia and tachypnea commonly occur. As shock progresses, these signs and symptoms appear: hypotension (systolic pressure of less than 80 mm Hg or 50 to 80 mm Hg less than the patient's baseline), thirst, anxiety, restlessness, and confusion. Pulse pressure narrows and the skin becomes cold, clammy, and cyanotic. The patient experiences oliguria or anuria, respiratory failure, and coma. His history may reveal conditions predisposing him to septic shock.

Other causes
In dialysis patients, a localized pulse absence may occur distal to arteriovenous shunts or fistulas.

Pulse pressure, narrowed

Pulse pressure, the difference between systolic and diastolic blood pressures, can be measured by sphygmomanometry or intra-arterial monitoring. Normally, systolic pressure exceeds diastolic pressure by about 40 mm Hg. Narrowed pulse pressure — a difference of less than 30 mm Hg — occurs when peripheral arterial resistance increases, cardiac output declines, or intravascular volume markedly decreases (see *Understanding pulse pressure changes*, page 142). In conditions that cause mechanical obstruction, such as aortic stenosis, pulse pressure is directly related to the severity of the underlying condition. Usually a late sign, narrowed pulse pressure alone doesn't signal an emergency, although it commonly occurs in shock.

History questions
Explore the patient's problem by asking appropriate questions from this section.
• Did a specific event precede the change in pulse pressure?
• Does the patient have an internal or external hemorrhage?
• Is he experiencing associated symptoms, such as itching, changes in level of consciousness, a feeling of impending doom, extreme thirst, nasal congestion, or urinary incontinence?
• Is he having any pain or discomfort, particularly headache, chest, or abdominal pain? If so, have him describe the pain. When did it start in relation to the pulse pressure change?
• Has he been exposed to any known or common allergens? Has he recently been stung by a bee or another insect? What about changes in his diet or physical environment?
• Does his recent history include chest trauma, pericarditis, myocardial infarction, fever, malaise, or chronic tamponade? Has he had a surgical procedure or immunosup-

PATHOPHYSIOLOGY

Understanding pulse pressure changes

Two major factors affect pulse pressure: the amount of blood that the ventricles eject into the arteries with each beat (*stroke volume*) and the arteries' *peripheral resistance* to blood flow. These two factors affect systolic and diastolic blood pressures and, as a result, pulse pressure. For example, pulse pressure narrows when systolic pressure falls and diastolic pressure remains constant, when diastolic pressure rises and systolic pressure stays constant, or when systolic pressure falls and diastolic pressure rises. These changes reflect reduced stroke volume, increased peripheral resistance, or both.

Pulse pressure widens when systolic pressure rises and diastolic pressure remains constant, when diastolic pressure falls and systolic pressure remains constant, or when systolic pressure rises and diastolic pressure falls. These changes reflect increased stroke volume, decreased peripheral resistance, or both.

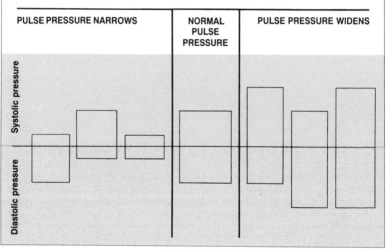

pressive therapy that could predispose him to infection?
• Is he taking any medications, such as penicillins or sulfonamides, that may cause anaphylaxis?

Physical examination
Base your assessment of the patient on the health history information you've collected.

Inspection. Observe the rate and depth of the patient's respirations. Does he have difficulty breathing or an abnormal respiratory pattern? Listen for any stridor or hoarseness, which suggests laryngeal edema.

As you inspect the patient's skin, look for urticaria, flushing, and cyanosis. Then assess his level of consciousness, noting any alterations, such as restlessness, lethargy, stupor, or coma. Inspect his neck for jugular vein distention. And monitor urine output for oliguria and anuria.

Palpation. Check for hepatomegaly. Also, palpate the peripheral pulses, noting their rate, rhythm, and intensity.

Percussion. Assess the patient's abdomen for hepatomegaly.

Auscultation. Monitor the patient's blood pressure and pulse pressure. As you auscultate blood pressure, note the intensity of Korotkoff's sounds. Do you detect pulsus paradoxus? Auscultate for heart sounds, listening particularly for any murmurs, gallops, or irregular heart rhythms. Auscultate the lungs for abnormal sounds.

Life-threatening causes

Your assessment may lead you to suspect one or more of the following.

Anaphylactic shock. In this disorder, a narrowed pulse pressure and a dramatic drop in blood pressure usually follow a rapid, weak pulse that soon becomes uniformly absent. Within seconds or minutes of exposure to an allergen, the patient experiences extreme anxiety, restlessness, and a feeling of doom, along with intense itching (especially of the hands and feet), a pounding headache, and possibly urticaria. (Keep in mind, however, that delayed reactions of up to 24 hours can occur.) Later, you may note dyspnea, stridor, coughing, and hoarseness from laryngeal edema, as well as nasal congestion, chest or throat tightness, cardiac dysrhythmias, tachycardia, skin flushing, nausea, abdominal cramps, urinary incontinence, and seizures. The patient may have allergies or a family history of them and have been exposed to a known or common allergen. For instance, he may have been stung by a bee or taken a drug such as a penicillin or sulfonamide.

Cardiac tamponade. Pulse pressure that narrows 10 to 20 mm Hg, jugular vein distention, hypotension, and muffled heart sounds are the classic signs of cardiac tamponade. However, a hypovolemic patient may not have jugular vein distention, and if a patient sits upright, his heart sounds may not be muffled. The patient may appear anxious and restless. He may also have chest pain, clammy skin, weak peripheral pulses, tachycardia, pulsus paradoxus, and dyspnea. Later, cyanosis can occur along with pericardial friction rubs and hepatomegaly. As you review the patient's history, you may find recent chest trauma, pericarditis, myocardial infarction, fever, malaise, or chronic tamponade.

Cardiogenic shock. In this disorder, narrowed pulse pressure is accompanied by a drop in systolic pressure to 30 mm Hg below baseline or a sustained reading below 80 mm Hg not caused by medication. Other signs and symptoms include absent peripheral pulses, weak central pulses, diminished Korotkoff's sounds, peripheral cyanosis from poor tissue perfusion, and cool, clammy skin. Poor tissue perfusion also causes restlessness and anxiety. The patient's signs and symptoms may progress to disorientation and confusion, anginal pain, dyspnea, jugular vein distention, and oliguria. On auscultation, you may detect tachypnea, tachycardia, faint heart sounds, ventricular gallop, and possibly a systolic murmur. The patient's history may include disorders that cause left ventricular dysfunction.

Hypovolemic shock. Narrowed pulse pressure will be accompanied by a fall in systolic blood pressure to less than 80 mm Hg or 30 mm Hg less than the patient's baseline. You may find orthostatic pressure changes, diminished Korotkoff's sounds, tachypnea and tachycardia that worsen as blood volume decreases, and a weak, occasionally irregular pulse. You may also note angina (in patients with coronary artery disease), light-headedness, irritability, diaphoresis, extreme thirst, hypothermia, oliguria, confusion, disorientation, restlessness, and anxiety. Peripheral vasoconstriction causes cyanosis of the limbs and pale, cool, clammy skin. The history may reveal a source of the volume loss.

Septic shock. In the late stage of septic shock, narrowed pulse pressure develops along with severe hypotension (less than 80 mm Hg or 50 to 80 mm Hg less than the patient's baseline). You may also note tachycardia; dysrhythmias; a weak, thready pulse; decreased or absent peripheral pulses; rapid, shallow respirations; a decreased level of consciousness, possibly progressing to coma; pale skin; cyanotic limbs; and oliguria or anuria from decreased cardiac output. The patient's history may include conditions predisposing him to septic shock.

Other causes

Narrowed pulse pressure also occurs in aortic stenosis.

***

Pulse pressure, widened

Widened pulse pressure — a difference of more than 50 mm Hg between systolic and diastolic blood pressures — commonly occurs as a physiologic response to fever, hot weather, or exercise. However, it can also result from certain neurologic and cardiovascular disorders that reduce arterial compliance or cause a backflow of blood into the heart with each contraction. Chief among these disorders is a life-threatening increase in intracranial pressure (ICP).

Widened pulse pressure can easily be identified by monitoring arterial blood pressure, and it's commonly detected during routine sphygmomanometric recordings.

History questions

Explore the patient's problem by asking appropriate questions from this section. If the patient is comatose, you'll have to obtain the necessary information from a family member, someone who brought the patient to the hospital, or the hospital record.

• Does the patient have other symptoms, such as an altered level of consciousness (LOC), bradycardia, hypertension, fever, or respiratory pattern changes? What about nausea, vertigo, or headache?

• If his LOC has changed, when did the change begin? Was it a slow or abrupt deterioration? Did a specific incident precede the onset of symptoms — a head injury, for instance?

• Has the patient recently been exposed to high temperatures or been exercising strenuously? Has he been exposed to poisonous substances?

• Does the patient have a history of endocrine, hepatic, renal, neurologic, or cardiovascular disease? How about cancer, anoxia, or electrolyte or acid-base imbalances? Does he have a history of drug or alcohol abuse?

Physical examination
Base your assessment of the patient on the health history information you've collected.

Inspection. Using the Glasgow Coma Scale, evaluate the patient's LOC (see *Using the Glasgow Coma Scale*, page 118). Also, check cranial nerve function, especially for cranial nerves III, IV, and VI. Assess his pupillary reactions. If a cervical spine injury has been ruled out, perform the doll's eye maneuver, noting eye movement and dysconjugate gaze.

Observe the rate and depth of his respirations. Do you note difficulty breathing or an abnormal respiratory pattern, such as Cheyne-Stokes or apneustic respirations, central neurogenic hyperventilation, ataxic respirations, or apnea?

Monitor the patient's urine output for oliguria or evidence of diabetes insipidus.

Palpation. Check the peripheral pulses for rate, rhythm, and intensity. Then palpate the muscles to assess if they're hypotonic or hypertonic.

Percussion. Stimulate the patient by exerting firm pressure on his nail beds or Achilles tendon, and note any posturing changes. Check deep tendon reflexes, watching for abnormal responses. Compare responses bilaterally.

Auscultation. Monitor the patient's blood pressure and pulse pressure.

Life-threatening cause
Your assessment may lead you to suspect this disorder.

Increased ICP. Widening pulse pressure is an intermediate to late sign of increased ICP. This danger sign may be accompanied by bradycardia, hypertension, and tachypnea or respiratory pattern changes. The onset and progression of widening pulse pressure parallel the rising ICP. A gap of just 50 mm Hg can signal a rapid deterioration in the patient's condition.

The earliest and most sensitive indicator of this condition, a decreased LOC may be accompanied by persistent headache, tachycardia, projectile vomiting, or seizures. Decorticate posture appears when ICP is elevated enough to compress the midbrain. This sign may be accompanied by fixed pupils that are at the midposition, absent doll's eye sign, dysconjugate gaze, Cheyne-Stokes respirations or central neurogenic hyperventilation, wide variations in body temperature, and diabetes insipidus. Decerebrate posture occurs when the increased pressure affects the pons. This sign is usually accompanied by small, fixed pupils; possibly doll's eye sign and dysconjugate gaze; central neurogenic hyperventilation or apneustic respirations; elevated temperature; and an erratic pulse. Progressive neurologic deterioration to the medulla causes ataxic respirations followed by apnea, flaccidity, and an absent pulse. Signs and symptoms of the underlying disorder may also be present. The patient's history may include a systemic or brain infection, head trauma, brain tumor, or underlying metabolic or cardiovascular disease.

Other causes
Widened pulse pressure commonly occurs as a physiologic response to fever, hot weather, and exercise. The sign also occurs in acute aortic insufficiency, arteriosclerosis, and patent ductus arteriosus.

Pulse rhythm abnormality

An irregular expansion and contraction of the peripheral arterial walls, abnormal pulse rhythm results from an irregular heartbeat. You may first detect this sign by palpating the radial or carotid pulse after a patient complains of palpitations. To effectively evaluate an abnormal pulse rhythm, you must auscultate the heart as you palpate one of these pulses.

History questions
Explore the patient's problem by asking appropriate questions from this section.
• Is the patient feeling chest pain, palpitations, dizziness, or weakness? What about muscle cramps or spasms in his feet or hands? Any numbness or tingling in his fingertips, feet, or mouth?
• Does the patient have a history of a cardiovascular or pulmonary disorder that could produce dysrhythmias?
• Is the patient taking any medications? If so, find out whether he's complying with the prescribed regimen. Particularly note any drugs that can cause dysrhythmias, including digitalis glycosides, sympathomimetics, ganglionic blockers, aminophylline, and atropine. Also, determine whether he uses caffeine, tobacco, marijuana, or alcohol.

Physical examination
Base your assessment of the patient on the health history information you've collected.

Inspection. Assess for a decreased level of consciousness (LOC) — an important sign of inadequate cerebral perfusion. Check the skin for pallor or diaphoresis, and inspect the fingertips for capillary nail bed pulsations. Assess the respiratory rate and depth, and note any difficulty breathing or abnormal respiratory patterns.

Palpation. Simultaneously palpate the radial or carotid artery and auscultate the apical pulse. Note any difference between the rates. Also, palpate the peripheral pulses, noting rate, rhythm, and intensity.

Auscultation. Next, evaluate the patient's heart sounds, listening for abnormal rhythms, gallops, or murmurs. Auscultate over the lungs to detect abnormal breath sounds. Be sure to monitor the patient's blood pressure and pulse pressure.

Life-threatening cause
Your assessment may lead you to suspect this cause.

Cardiac dysrhythmias. An abnormal pulse rhythm may be the only indication of a cardiac dysrhythmia, or the patient may complain of palpitations or a fluttering heartbeat. Depending on the specific dysrhythmia, dull chest pain or discomfort and hypotension also may occur. Associated findings reflect decreased cardiac output; these may include confusion, dizziness, lightheadedness, decreased LOC, seizures, decreased urine output, dyspnea, tachypnea, pallor, and diaphoresis. The patient's history may include cardiac or pulmonary disease, sepsis, electrolyte imbalance, or use of drugs that can cause dysrhythmias.

Other causes
Certain causes of pulse rhythm abnormality may not signal the need

for immediate intervention.

Disorders. Among the disorders that can cause abnormal pulse rhythm are acute anxiety attack, anemia, aortic insufficiency, hypertension, hypoglycemia, mitral prolapse, mitral stenosis, mitral regurgitation, and pheochromocytoma. Other contributing factors include physical and emotional stress. In children and young adults, you may palpate sinus arrhythmia — a normal rhythm variation.

Drugs. Abnormal pulse rhythm may result from drugs that precipitate cardiac dysrhythmias or increase cardiac output, such as digitalis glycosides, sympathomimetics, ganglionic blockers, aminophylline, and atropine. Caffeine, tobacco, marijuana, or alcohol also can precipitate minor rhythm abnormalities.

Surgery. Abnormal pulse rhythm may occur after coronary bypass or valve replacement surgery.

Pulsus alternans

A sign of severe left ventricular failure, pulsus alternans is a beat-to-beat change in the intensity of a peripheral pulse. Although the pulse rhythm remains regular, you'll note alternating strong and weak contractions (see *Comparing arterial pressure waves,* page 148). This sign may be accompanied by heart sounds and heart murmurs that alternate in intensity.

Pulsus alternans is thought to result from the changes in stroke volume that occur with beat-to-beat changes in left ventricular contractility. Lying down or exercising

How to detect pulsus alternans

Using a sphygmomanometer is the easiest way to detect pulsus alternans. But when systolic pressure varies from beat to beat by more than 20 mm Hg, you can also detect this sign by palpating the brachial, radial, or femoral artery. Sometimes, the small changes in arterial pressure that occur during normal respirations can obscure the abnormal pulse. So ask the patient to hold his breath as you palpate. Also, be sure to apply only *light* pressure to avoid obliterating the weaker pulse.

Occasionally, you won't be able to detect the weak beat when you're palpating a patient's peripheral pulse. This is known as total pulsus alternans, an apparent halving of the pulse rate.

When using a sphygmomanometer to detect pulsus alternans, inflate the cuff 10 to 20 mm Hg above the systolic pressure as determined by palpation. Then slowly deflate the cuff. At first, you'll hear only the strong beats. With further deflation, all beats will become audible and palpable, and then equally intense. The difference between the reading at this point and the systolic reading is commonly used to determine the degree of pulsus alternans. When you remove the cuff, pulsus alternans will return.

increases venous return and reduces the abnormal pulse. Often, this sign disappears with treatment for left ventricular failure.

You can detect pulsus alternans by using a sphygmomanometer or by palpating the brachial, radial, or femoral pulse (see *How to detect pulsus alternans*).

History questions
Explore the patient's problem by

Comparing arterial pressure waves

These three graphs illustrate the differences among normal arterial pulse, pulsus alternans, and pulsus paradoxus. The shaded area indicates the inspiratory phase of respiration; the unshaded area, the expiratory phase.

Normal arterial pulse

The percussion wave in the normal arterial pulse reflects ejection of blood into the aorta (early systole). The tidal wave is the peak of the pulse wave (later systole). And the dicrotic notch marks the beginning of diastole.

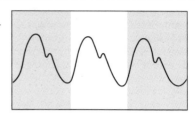

Pulsus alternans

This beat-to-beat alternation in pulse size and intensity has a regular rhythm but a variable volume. If you take the blood pressure of a patient with this abnormality, you'll first hear a loud Korotkoff's sound and then a soft sound, continually alternating. Pulsus alternans frequently accompanies states of poor contractility that occur with left ventricular failure.

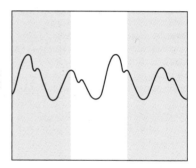

Pulsus paradoxus

An exaggerated decline in blood pressure during inspiration, pulsus paradoxus results from an increase in negative intrathoracic pressure. Considered abnormal, pulsus paradoxus may indicate cardiac tamponade, constrictive pericarditis, or severe lung disease.

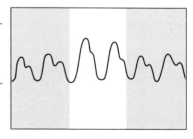

asking appropriate questions from this section.
• Does the patient have trouble breathing when he lies down or increases his activity? Does he wake up during the night feeling breathless? Has he experienced fatigue, weakness, or recent weight gain?

Does he have a productive cough? If so, have him describe the color and characteristics of the sputum.
• Does the patient have a history of a disorder that could progress to left ventricular failure?
• What medications is the patient taking? Note whether he's taking

any drugs that may predispose him to congestive heart failure — beta-blockers, for example.

Physical examination
Base your assessment of the patient on the health history information you've collected.

Inspection. Observe the rate and depth of the patient's respirations. Do you note any difficulty breathing or abnormal respiratory patterns? Inspect his skin and mucous membranes for cyanosis, edema, and diaphoresis. Then assess his nail beds for prolonged capillary refill time and look for jugular vein distention.

Also, determine the patient's level of consciousness and monitor him for changes, such as anxiety and restlessness, which can indicate decreased cerebral perfusion.

Palpation. Evaluate the rate, rhythm, and intensity of the peripheral pulses. Then, palpate the arms and legs for pitting edema, and the abdomen for hepatomegaly.

Percussion. Gently percuss the abdomen to detect hepatomegaly.

Auscultation. Evaluate heart sounds, noting any murmurs, ventricular gallops, or continually alternating loud and soft Korotkoff's sounds. Then, auscultate all lung fields for adventitious sounds, particularly crackles and rhonchi.

Life-threatening cause
Your assessment may lead you to suspect this cause.

Left ventricular failure. In this disorder, pulsus alternans is often initiated by a premature beat. This sign is almost always associated with a ventricular gallop. Other findings may include alternating loud and soft Korotkoff's sounds, tachycardia, hypotension, and pallor or cyanosis. Respiratory findings may include Cheyne-Stokes respirations, nocturnal dyspnea, tachypnea, and bilateral crackles. Fatigue and weakness are common. You also may detect jugular vein distention, prolonged capillary refill time, dependent edema, hepatomegaly, diaphoresis, and anxiety. If the patient has an associated cough, it'll usually be nonproductive. However, a patient may develop a cough that produces clear or blood-tinged sputum. Typically, the patient's history reveals cardiac disease accompanied by atherosclerosis.

Other cause
Rarely, pulsus alternans occurs in a patient with normal left ventricular function and doesn't indicate an underlying disorder. In such a patient, the abnormal pulse seldom persists for more than 10 to 12 beats.

Pulsus paradoxus

A classic sign of cardiac tamponade, pulsus paradoxus (also called paradoxical pulse) is an exaggerated blood pressure drop during inspiration. Normally, systolic pressure falls less than 10 mm Hg during inspiration. In pulsus paradoxus, it falls more than 10 mm Hg. (See *Comparing arterial pressure waves.*) When systolic pressure falls more than 20 mm Hg, the peripheral pulses may be barely palpable, or they may disappear during inspiration.

Pulsus paradoxus apparently

How to detect paradoxical pulse

To accurately detect and measure paradoxical pulse, you can use a sphygmomanometer and stethoscope. First, inflate the blood pressure cuff 10 to 20 mm Hg beyond the peak systolic pressure. Then, deflate the cuff at a rate of 2 mm Hg/second until you hear the first Korotkoff's sound during expiration; note the systolic pressure.

As you continue slowly deflating the cuff, observe the patient's respiratory pattern. If he has a paradoxical pulse, Korotkoff's sounds will cease on inspiration and return on expiration.

Continue deflating the cuff until you hear Korotkoff's sounds during both inspiration and expiration, and, again, note the systolic pressure.

Now subtract the second reading from the first reading. A difference between the readings of more than 10 mm Hg indicates that the patient has a paradoxical pulse.

You also can detect paradoxical pulse by palpating the radial pulse over several cycles of slow inspiration and expiration. A marked pulse decrease during inspiration indicates paradoxical pulse.

When assessing for paradoxical pulse, remember that irregular heart rhythms and tachycardia can also cause variations in pulse amplitude. So rule out these possibilities before determining that your patient has a paradoxical pulse.

stems from an inspirational increase in negative intrathoracic pressure. Normally, systolic pressure drops during inspiration because of blood pooling in the pulmonary system. This pooling, in turn, reduces left ventricular filling and stroke volume and transmits negative intrathoracic pressure to the aorta. Conditions that further impede blood flow from

the left ventricle during inspiration, such as chronic obstructive pulmonary disease (COPD) or cardiac tamponade, can produce pulsus paradoxus.

You can accurately detect and measure a paradoxical pulse with a sphygmomanometer or an intra-arterial pressure monitoring device. You can also detect this sign by palpating the radial pulse. (For more information, see *How to detect paradoxical pulse.*)

History questions

Explore the patient's problem by asking appropriate questions from this section.

• Is the patient experiencing associated signs or symptoms, such as chest pain, dyspnea, or cough? If he reports chest pain, have him describe its onset, severity, character, and location. Is the pain aggravated by inspiration or movement? If he complains of dyspnea, determine whether it started suddenly or gradually. If he reports a productive cough, ask about the amount and character of sputum produced.

• Does the patient have a history of cardiovascular disease, particularly hypertension, myocardial infarction (MI), pericarditis, congestive heart failure (CHF), or cardiomyopathy? What about hypercholesterolemia, thrombophlebitis, or varicose veins? Has he sustained chest trauma or a recent hip or leg fracture?

• If the patient is a woman, is she pregnant? Is she in the postpartum period? Does she take oral contraceptives?

• Has the patient recently undergone insertion of a central venous catheter, pulmonary artery catheter, or a temporary transvenous or permanent pacemaker?

• Is the patient taking any medications? Note anticoagulant use.

Physical examination

Base your assessment of the patient on the health history information you've collected.

Inspection. Observe the patient's respiratory effort. Is he tachypneic or dyspneic? Note his posture: Is he leaning forward in an attempt to breathe more easily? Also, look for signs of poor cerebral perfusion, such as restlessness, confusion, or seizures.

Inspect the skin for diaphoresis or central or peripheral cyanosis. Look too for jugular vein distention. If the patient coughs, assess any sputum produced. To detect oliguria, monitor the patient's urine output.

Palpation. Assess the intensity, rate, and rhythm of all peripheral pulses. Then palpate the abdomen to locate the liver and check for hepatomegaly.

Evaluate the abdominojugular reflex: Place your palm firmly on the right upper abdominal quadrant and apply moderate pressure for 30 seconds. Observe for an increasingly visible jugular pulse.

Percussion. Gently percuss the abdomen, evaluating the liver for hepatomegaly. Also, percuss over the lungs, noting areas of dullness.

Auscultation. As you auscultate blood pressure, note the decrease in systolic pressure when the patient inhales and the narrowed pulse pressure. Evaluate heart sounds, checking for muffled sounds, systolic murmur, tricuspid regurgitation, tachycardia, or pericardial friction rubs. Auscultate along the left sternal border for an S_3 or S_4. If you detect one of these sounds, does it intensify on inspiration? Auscultate the lungs to detect decreased breath sounds, crackles, diffuse wheezing, or pleural friction rubs.

Life-threatening causes

Your assessment may lead you to suspect one or more of the following.

Cardiac tamponade. A classic finding in cardiac tamponade, pulsus paradoxus is typically accompanied by jugular vein distention, hypotension, narrowed pulse pressure, and muffled heart sounds. However, pulsus paradoxus may be difficult to detect if intrapericardial pressure rises abruptly and profound hypotension develops. Common associated signs and symptoms include chest pain, pericardial friction rubs, anxiety, restlessness, fever, malaise, clammy skin, and hepatomegaly. Characteristic respiratory findings include dyspnea, tachypnea, and cyanosis. The patient typically sits up and leans forward to ease breathing. His history may reveal chronic tamponade or recent chest trauma, pericarditis, or MI.

Pulmonary embolism. With massive pulmonary embolism, decreased left ventricular filling and stroke volume commonly cause pulsus paradoxus. Syncope, severe apprehension, sudden dyspnea, tachypnea, and an abrupt onset of angina-like or pleuritic pain may also occur. Typically, the patient appears cyanotic with jugular vein distention. Other findings may include tachycardia, hypotension, restlessness, diaphoresis, crackles, wheezing, low-grade fever, and dullness on chest percussion.

An infarction may produce hemoptysis, along with decreased breath sounds and a pleural friction rub over the affected area. The patient may also show signs of cerebral ischemia, such as transient unconsciousness, coma, seizures, and, particularly in an elderly patient, hemiplegia and other focal neurologic deficits. The patient's history may reveal thrombophlebitis of the deep systemic veins, varicose veins, hip or leg fracture, acute MI, CHF, cardiogenic shock, congestive cardiomyopathy, pregnancy, or oral contraceptive use.

Right ventricular infarction. The patient may have pulsus paradoxus and elevated jugular or central venous pressure, along with the classic signs and symptoms of MI. You may also detect S_3 and S_4 at the left sternal border that intensify on inspiration, a systolic murmur of tricuspid regurgitation, a positive abdominojugular reflex, hepatomegaly, and peripheral edema. He may show signs of shock (hypotension, tachycardia, weak or absent pulses, peripheral cyanosis, restlessness, anxiety, oliguria, and cool, clammy skin) with no evidence of pulmonary congestion. His history may reveal cardiac disease, hypertension, or hypercholesterolemia.

Other causes
Paradoxical pulse also results from conditions that may not require immediate intervention. For instance, you may detect this sign in a patient with COPD or chronic constrictive pericarditis. It also commonly occurs in children with chronic pulmonary disease, particularly during acute asthma attacks.

Pupillary changes

A change in pupil size, equality, or reactivity may indicate a serious neurologic problem. Commonly, pupils are described as dilated, midsized, or pinpoint. But by measuring pupil size in millimeters, you can monitor the patient more precisely and thus detect small but significant changes.

Normally, both pupils constrict equally when exposed to light and dilate when the light is removed. An abnormal pupillary reaction (or reflex) may be unilateral or bilateral and can indicate dysfunction of cranial nerves II and III, a brain tumor, increased intracranial pressure (ICP), or brain stem damage. (For more information, see *Understanding direct and consensual light reflexes.*) When you test reactivity to light, you'll describe the pupils as reactive, sluggish, or nonreactive (also referred to as fixed).

As you examine the patient, keep in mind that pupil size and reactivity may be affected by certain drugs or a previous eye injury. So note the patient's condition and check his health history before deciding that pupillary changes are significant.

History questions
Explore the patient's problem by asking appropriate questions from this section.
• Are the patient's pupils normally equal in size? How do they normally react to light?
• Is he experiencing any pain? If so, determine its location, intensity, and duration. Also, ask about associated signs and symptoms, such as headache, nausea, and vomiting. When did these symptoms develop? Did they begin gradually or suddenly? If he has a headache, has it been getting worse? If he's vomiting, is it projectile?
• Has he noticed a visual disturbance, such as blurred or double vision, photophobia, or decreased

Understanding direct and consensual light reflexes

Two reactions—direct and consensual—constitute the pupillary light reflex. Normally, shining a light directly onto the retina of one eye stimulates the parasympathetic nerves to cause brisk constriction of that pupil—the *direct light reflex*. The pupil of the opposite eye also constricts—the *consensual light reflex*.

The optic nerve (cranial nerve II) mediates the afferent arc of this reflex from each eye, while the oculomotor nerve (cranial nerve III) mediates the efferent arc to both eyes. A nonreactive or sluggish response in one or both pupils indicates dysfunction of these cranial nerves—usually from degenerative disease of the central nervous system.

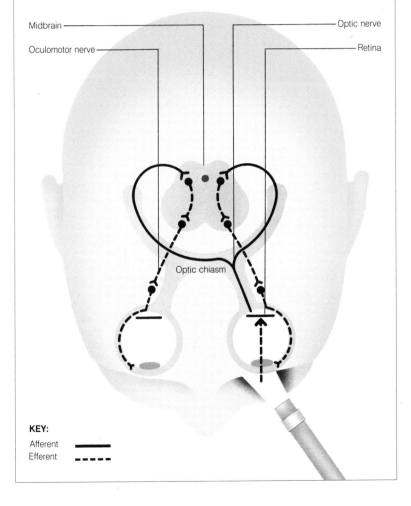

Midbrain

Oculomotor nerve

Optic nerve

Retina

Optic chiasm

KEY:

Afferent ▬▬▬▬

Efferent ▬ ▬ ▬ ▬

Assessing pupillary reflexes

To assess pupillary reaction to light, first test the patient's *direct light reflex.* Darken the room, and cover one of the patient's eyes while you hold open the opposite eye. Using a bright penlight, bring the light toward the patient from the side and shine it directly into her opened eye. If normal, the pupil will promptly constrict.

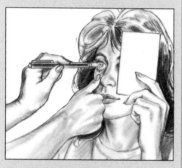

Now, test the *consensual light reflex.* Hold the patient's eyes open and shine the light into one eye while watching the pupil of the opposite eye. If normal, both pupils will promptly constrict.

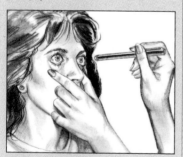

Repeat both procedures on the patient's other eye, and compare your findings. A unilateral or bilateral nonreactive response indicates dysfunction of cranial nerves II and III, which mediate the pupillary light reflex.

acuity? Does he see halos around lights at night (halo vision)?
• Has the patient suffered a head injury? If so, ask about the cause and nature of it. Also, investigate any episodes of unconsciousness or seizures. Was the unconsciousness followed by a lucid period? When did seizures occur in relation to the unconsciousness?
• Does the patient wear an eye prosthesis? Does he have a systemic or brain infection, brain tumor, or cardiovascular or metabolic disease? Has he recently undergone brain surgery? Has an ophthalmologic examination revealed glaucoma or increased intraocular pressure?
• What medications is the patient taking? Is he using eyedrops? If so, when did he last instill them? Has he recently received atropine or an opiate, such as morphine? Does he use any street drugs or tobacco?

Physical examination
Base your assessment of the patient on the health history information you've collected.

Inspection. Note the size of the patient's pupils and test their reaction to light (see *Assessing pupillary reflexes* and *Understanding pupillary changes*). Check for downward deviation of the eyes, uncontrolled movements, conjunctival injection, or swelling of the eyelids. Then examine the cornea and iris for any abnormalities, such as corneal clouding, and assess the visual acuity of both eyes. Also, test the patient's pupillary accommodation. Normally, both pupils constrict equally as the patient shifts his glance from a distant to a near object.

Now, assess level of consciousness (LOC) and monitor for any changes. Observe body position and move-

Understanding pupillary changes

Use this chart as a guide to the significance of pupillary changes.

PUPILLARY CHANGE	POSSIBLE CAUSES
Unilateral, dilated (4 mm), fixed, and non-reactive 	• Uncal herniation with oculomotor nerve damage • Brain stem compression from an expanding lesion or an aneurysm • Increased intracranial pressure • Tentorial herniation • Head trauma with subsequent subdural or epidural hematoma • May be normal in some people
Bilateral, dilated (4 mm), fixed, and nonreactive 	• Severe midbrain damage • Cardiopulmonary arrest (hypoxia) • Anticholinergic poisoning
Bilateral, mid-sized (2 mm), fixed, and nonreactive 	• Midbrain involvement caused by edema, hemorrhage, infarctions, lacerations, contusions
Bilateral, pinpoint (less than 1 mm), and usually nonreactive 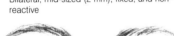	• Lesion of pons, usually after hemorrhage, leading to blocked sympathetic impulses • Opiates, such as morphine (pupils may be reactive)
Unilateral, small (1.5 mm), and nonreactive 	• Disruption of sympathetic nerve supply to the head caused by spinal cord lesion above T1

ments, noting seizures, paresis, paralysis, and decerebrate or decorticate posture. Check also for positive Kernig's and Babinski's signs.

As you observe the patient, note any abnormal respiratory patterns, such as Cheyne-Stokes respirations, apneustic breathing, or central neurogenic hyperventilation.

To check for oliguria and evidence of diabetes insipidus, monitor the patient's urine output.

Palpation. Estimate intraocular pressure by placing your fingers over the patient's closed eyelid. If the eyeball feels rock-hard, suspect elevated intraocular pressure. Next, palpate all peripheral pulses, noting rate, rhythm, and intensity. When touching the patient, note any diaphoresis or loss of sensation.

Percussion. Test the patient's deep tendon reflexes.

Auscultation. Monitor the patient's blood pressure and pulse pressure.

Life- or vision-threatening causes

Your assessment may lead you to suspect one or more of the following.

Brain herniation. In this disorder, the patient has a unilaterally dilated, nonreactive pupil. Initially, the pupil may appear oval-shaped, indicating intracranial hypertension. Related findings include a diminished LOC, hypertension, bradycardia, widening pulse pressure, an altered respiratory pattern, diminished sensory function, hemiparesis, hemiplegia, headache, and vomiting. The patient may have a history of a systemic infection, head trauma, brain surgery, brain tumor, or underlying metabolic disease.

Cerebral aneurysm (ruptured). Depending on the site and severity of the hemorrhage, the patient may have bilateral miotic but reactive pupils accompanied by an altered LOC, possibly leading to coma. Deep coma occurs with severe bleeding. In most cases, these signs immediately follow an abrupt onset of excruciating headache, nausea, and vomiting. Meningeal irritation may produce nuchal rigidity, back and leg pain, fever, restlessness, irritability, seizures, and blurred vision. Other findings may include hemiparesis, hemisensory deficit, dysphagia, gait ataxia, visual defects, and downward deviation of the eye or conjugate deviation of the eye toward the affected side. The patient's history may include hypertension or other cardiovascular disorders, a stressful life-style, smoking, or excessive caffeine intake.

Cerebral contusion. Severe cerebral injury can produce dilated, nonreactive pupils along with a sudden or gradual decrease in LOC. The patient may be unconscious for a prolonged period or, if conscious, he may be drowsy, confused, disoriented, agitated, or even violent. He may also experience blurred or double vision, fever, headache, pallor, diaphoresis, tachycardia, altered respirations, aphasia, hemiparesis, and decorticate or decerebrate posture. Common residual effects include seizures, impaired mental status, slight hemiparesis, and vertigo. The health history will include recent head trauma (which the patient may not reveal in a case of physical abuse).

Epidural hemorrhage (acute). Ipsilateral pupil dilation commonly accompanies an immediate, brief loss of consciousness that's followed by a lucid interval in 30% to 40% of patients. Related findings include a rapid, steady decline in LOC and a progressively severe headache. You may also note vomiting, unilateral seizures, contralateral hemiparesis, hemiplegia, high fever, and signs of increasing ICP. The patient's history typically includes head trauma within the past 24 hours.

Glaucoma (acute closed-angle.) With this disorder, which endangers your patient's eyesight, you'll see a moderately dilated, fixed pupil in the affected eye. You'll also note conjunctival injection, corneal clouding, decreased visual acuity, hardened eyeball, and swollen upper eyelid. The patient likely will report blurred vision that developed suddenly, followed by excruciating pain in and around the affected eye and a generalized headache. He also may complain of other visual disturbances such as halo vision and photophobia. Nausea and vomiting may indicate severely elevated intraocular pressure. The patient may have a history of chronic glaucoma, elevated intraocular pressure, or progressive vision blurring.

Increased ICP. As ICP increases, the patient develops a dilated, fixed pupil along with other signs and symptoms of progressive neurologic deterioration. The onset may be gradual or sudden. Earlier findings typically include elevated blood pressure, bradycardia, widened pulse pressure, altered mentation, progressive loss of consciousness, persistent headache, projectile vomiting, and seizures. The patient may also have signs and symptoms of the underlying disorder. His health history may include systemic

or brain infection, head trauma, brain tumor, or underlying metabolic or cardiovascular disease.

Midbrain lesions. These lesions produce bilateral midposition, fixed pupils accompanied by absent doll's eye sign, and dysconjugate gaze. Decorticate posturing results from increased ICP on the midbrain. The patient will be comatose and may exhibit Cheyne-Stokes respirations or central neurogenic hyperventilation. Other common findings include widely fluctuating body temperature, bradycardia, hemiparesis or hemiplegia, and, possibly, diabetes insipidus. Common health history findings include systemic or brain infection, head trauma, brain tumor, or underlying metabolic or cardiovascular disease.

Pontine lesions. Compression of the pons from increased ICP typically produces small, fixed pupils possibly accompanied by absent doll's eye sign, dysconjugate gaze, and decerebrate posturing. Common associated findings include central neurogenic hyperventilation or apneustic respirations, elevated temperature, erratic pulse, total paralysis, and a positive Babinski's reflex. Pontine hemorrhage causes a sudden, rapid decrease in LOC that quickly progresses to coma and death. The patient's history may indicate systemic or brain infection, head trauma, brain tumor, or underlying metabolic or cardiovascular disease.

Subarachnoid hemorrhage. In this brain hemorrhage, ipsilateral pupil dilation occurs with a decreasing LOC that may rapidly progress to coma. Other effects include sudden violent headache, dizziness, photophobia, blurred vision, nausea and vomiting, hypertension, nuchal rigidity, and seizures. You may note positive Kernig's and Brudzinski's signs, fever, and focal neurologic effects such as hemiparesis, hemiplegia, sensory disturbances, and aphasia, along with other signs of elevated ICP. The patient may have a history of congenital vascular defects or arteriovenous malformation. Or his history may reveal underlying cardiovascular disease, smoking, excessive caffeine intake, or a stressful life-style.

Subdural hematoma (acute). This disorder commonly produces ipsilateral pupillary dilation progressing to fixation. Other early findings include severe, localized headache, which typically follows recent head trauma and an altered LOC, possibly progressing to somnolence and coma. Later, the patient may develop other signs of increased ICP and focal neurologic deficits, such as hemiparesis. The health history may reveal head trauma occurring within 3 days of the onset of symptoms, but about 50% of patients with subdural hematoma have no history of head trauma.

Other causes
Certain causes of pupillary changes may not require immediate intervention.

Disorders. A sluggish pupillary response can result from diabetic neuropathy, herpes zoster, acute iritis, multiple sclerosis, myotonic dystrophy, and tertiary syphilis. Nonreactive pupils may occur in botulism, degenerative or inflammatory iris disease, ocular trauma, oculomotor nerve palsy, and uveitis. A sluggish or nonreactive pupillary response can also occur in patients with familial amyloid polyneuropa-

thy, Adie's syndrome, or Wernicke's disease. Fright, sudden emotion, and hysteria can cause mydriasis.

Drugs. Instilling topical mydriatics and cycloplegics may induce a temporarily nonreactive pupil in the affected eye. Deep, ether-induced anesthesia or glutethimide produces medium-sized or slightly enlarged pupils, which remain nonreactive for several hours. Opiates, such as heroin and morphine, cause pinpoint pupils and a minimal light response that can be seen only with a magnifying glass. Atropine causes mydriasis, and anticholinergic poisoning produces widely dilated, nonreactive pupils.

Scrotal pain

In most cases, scrotal pain indicates a problem in the testes, epididymis, or vas deferens. But such pain can also be referred from other areas — the abdomen or kidneys, for instance.

By identifying the pain of testicular torsion early, you can prevent loss of the testes from ischemia.

History questions
Explore the patient's problem by asking appropriate questions from this section.
• When did the patient first notice the pain? Has it gotten progressively worse? Is he feeling any associated abdominal pain or nausea?
• Did the patient recently experience trauma to the scrotum or lower urinary tract?

Physical examination
Base your assessment of the patient

on the health history information you've collected. Be sure to auscultate the abdomen before palpating and percussing. Using this alternative sequence ensures that you don't affect the frequency or intensity of bowel sounds before you auscultate them.

Inspection. Observe the scrotum for bruising, swelling, and redness. Also, check the buttocks beneath the scrotum for bruising and the urethra for bleeding. Then, inspect the abdomen and costovertebral angle for evidence of trauma.

Auscultation. Next, auscultate the abdomen for diminished bowel sounds.

Palpation. Gently palpate the testicles, noting severe pain or tenderness. If you detect crepitus, urine may be collecting beneath the skin. Also, palpate the abdomen for pain or tenderness.

Percussion. Now, percuss the abdomen and flank for pain or tenderness.

Organ-threatening cause
Your assessment may lead you to suspect this cause.

Testicular torsion. In this acute disorder, scrotal pain develops rapidly and may be accompanied by abdominal pain and nausea. On palpating the testicles, you'll detect swelling and tenderness. The scrotum may appear discolored. The patient's history may reveal no predisposing factors. In many cases, this disorder occurs around puberty.

Other causes
Scrotal pain results from certain conditions that may not require im-

mediate intervention. These conditions include epididymitis, acute orchitis, scrotal burns, blunt scrotal trauma, spermatocele, and torsion of a hydatid of Morgagni. Pain caused by abdominal trauma, renal trauma, and urinary tract calculi may be referred to the scrotum.

Seizure, generalized tonic-clonic

A generalized tonic-clonic (or grand mal) seizure reflects the paroxysmal, uncontrolled discharge of central nervous system (CNS) neurons, leading to neurologic dysfunction. Unlike most other types of seizures, this cerebral hyperactivity isn't confined to a localized area but extends to the entire brain. The seizure typically begins with a prodrome, which may include an aura. As seizure activity spreads to the subcortical structures, the patient loses consciousness, falls to the ground, and may utter a loud cry that's precipitated by air rushing from the lungs through the vocal cords. His body stiffens (tonic phase), then undergoes rapid, synchronous muscle jerking and hyperventilation (clonic phase). The seizure usually stops after 2 to 5 minutes, when abnormal conduction of neurons stops. (See *Seizure stages,* page 160, and *How a seizure develops,* page 162.)

Generalized tonic-clonic seizures occur singly and can strike when the patient is awake and active or sleeping. If you witness the beginning of a seizure, you'll need to take appropriate steps to protect the patient from injury and prevent his airway from becoming obstructed

Seizure stages

Prodrome
This stage may include myoclonic jerks, a throbbing headache, or mood changes starting several hours or days before the seizure itself.

Aura
Also occurring before the seizure, an aura may include palpitations, epigastric distress rapidly rising to the throat, head or eye turning, and sensory hallucinations. Not all patients have auras.

Loss of consciousness
The patient loses consciousness as a sudden, intense electrical discharge overwhelms the brain's subcortical center.

Tonic phase
This stage lasts about 10 to 20 seconds. The patient's skeletal muscles contract and his body stiffens (see illustration). His eyelids open, arms flex, and legs extend. His mouth opens wide, then snaps shut. Respirations cease, leading to cyanosis. The patient arches his back and slowly lowers his arms. He may have fixed, dilated pupils and show a great increase in heart rate, blood pressure, salivation, tracheobronchial secretions, and diaphoresis.

Clonic phase
Lasting about 60 seconds, this phase starts with mild trembling and progresses to violent contractures or jerks (see illustration). The patient may grimace and spew foamy, bloody saliva. As the jerks quiet, the patient will still be apneic and unresponsive. He may have stertorous respirations and incontinence.

Recovery (postictal phase)
Level of consciousness increases after about 5 minutes, leaving the patient confused and disoriented. Muscle tone, heart rate, and blood pressure return to normal. He may sleep for several hours, awakening sore and exhausted.

TONIC PHASE

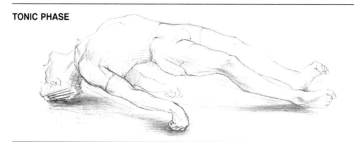

CLONIC PHASE

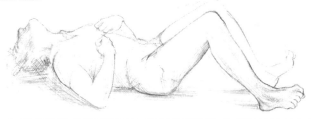

(see *When your patient has a seizure,* page 164). Possible complications include respiratory arrest caused by airway obstruction from secretions, status epilepticus (occurring in 5% to 8% of patients), head or spinal injuries and bruises, Todd's paralysis and, rarely, cardiac arrest.

History questions

When the patient is reoriented, explore his problem by asking appropriate questions from this section. If you didn't see the seizure occur, get a description of it from someone who did.

• When did the seizure start and how long did it last? Did it start in one area and spread, or did it affect the entire body right away?

• Did the patient feel any unusual sensations before the seizure? Also ask about emotional or physical stress at the time the seizure occurred.

• Find out about any associated signs and symptoms, such as nausea, vomiting, or diarrhea. Is the patient in pain? If so, have him describe the pain's onset, location, duration, and intensity. Does he have any visual disturbances, such as blurred vision, photophobia, impaired visual acuity, diplopia, or partial or total vision loss? Is he experiencing any muscle weakness, paralysis, or paresis? Any numbness or tingling of the arms or legs?

• Has the patient ever had generalized or focal seizures before? Are they frequent? Do other family members also have them? Has a doctor prescribed medication to control the seizures? Does the patient take it regularly?

• Investigate the patient's recent health history, particularly noting any head injury, infection, or exposure to viruses or bacteria known

to cause encephalitis or meningitis. Has he had any dental work done recently? What about recent or chronic exposure to pesticides containing arsenic or to substances containing lead?

• If the patient is pregnant, has she experienced sudden weight gain or generalized edema? Has she experienced pregnancy-induced hypertension during a previous pregnancy?

• If the patient is a child, has he recently had influenza, chicken pox, or a high fever? Does he live in an old building that has paint containing lead?

• Does the patient have a history of cardiovascular, metabolic, endocrine, hematologic, hepatic, or renal disease?

Physical examination

Base your assessment of the patient on the health history information you've collected.

Inspection. If you witness the seizure, note when it starts and how long it lasts. Also, note in which part of the body it starts, where it spreads, and whether it affects the entire body right away.

After the seizure, assess the patient's level of consciousness (LOC), noting such changes as irritability, restlessness, stupor, or coma. Observe the patient for decerebrate, decorticate, or opisthotonos posture. Note the rate and depth of his respirations. Does he have difficulty breathing? What about abnormal breathing patterns that may indicate neurologic damage—such as Cheyne-Stokes or apneustic respirations?

Check the patient's mouth for mucous membrane irritation and lead lines along the gums. Also, note any garlicky, fruity, or other unusual breath odor. Inspect the skin

PATHOPHYSIOLOGY

How a seizure develops

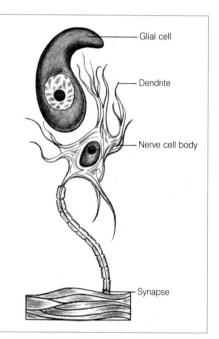

A seizure results from a disturbance in the depolarization-repolarization cycle caused by this sequence of events:
• The glial cell fails to keep the extracellular potassium level down.
• At the dendrite, the resulting potassium leakage leads to abnormal excitability.
• Then, in the nerve cell body, abnormal membrane permeability leads to a defect in the pumping mechanism, causing depolarization.
• At the synapse, repetitive after-discharge stimulation causes abnormal "reverse activation."

Glial cell

Dendrite

Nerve cell body

Synapse

---

for generalized or peripheral edema; diaphoresis; hyperpigmentation; hyperkeratosis; scaly, dry rash; pruritus; cold, clammy skin; decreased turgor; alopecia; and evidence of trauma. As you're inspecting the skin, note any trembling or muscle twitching.

Check the head and face for periorbital edema, facial muscle weakness, and signs of trauma. Look for nuchal rigidity and test for Brudzinski's and Kernig's signs. Be sure to inspect the pupils for equality and light reflex. Note any nystagmus.

Then monitor urine output to detect oliguria or anuria.

Palpation. Next, palpate peripheral

pulses, noting the rate, rhythm, and intensity. Gently palpate the patient's head to detect any changes in the normally hard, bony surface. Also, palpate the abdomen for pain.

Percussion. Assess deep tendon reflexes, noting any abnormal responses. Gently percuss the abdomen for pain or tenderness.

Auscultation. Carefully monitor blood pressure and pulse pressure.

Life-threatening causes
Your assessment may lead you to suspect one or more of the following.

Arsenic poisoning. Along with generalized seizures, arsenic poisoning commonly produces garlicky breath odor, increased salivation, generalized pruritus, diarrhea, nausea, vomiting, and severe abdominal pain. The patient rapidly develops cardiovascular collapse and shock. Related effects of chronic exposure may include diffuse hyperpigmentation; hyperkeratosis; scaly, dry rash; transverse white lines in the fingernails; sharply defined edema of the eyelids, face, and ankles; alopecia; mucous membrane irritation; weakness; muscle aches; and peripheral neuropathy. The patient's history will include arsenic ingestion or, rarely, exposure to pesticides containing arsenic.

Brain abscess. Generalized seizures may occur in the acute stage of abscess formation or after the abscess resolves. Depending on the size and location of the abscess, decreased LOC varies from drowsiness to deep stupor. Early signs and symptoms reflect increased intracranial pressure (ICP) and include constant headache, nausea, vomiting, and focal seizures. Typical later features include ocular disturbances such as nystagmus, impaired visual acuity, and unequal pupils. Other findings depend on the abscess site and may include aphasia, ataxia, hemiparesis, and behavioral and personality changes. Signs of infection, such as fever and pallor, may develop late; they may not develop at all if the abscess remains encapsulated, as it does in about 50% of cases. Typically, the patient will have a history of infection (systemic, chronic middle ear, mastoid, or sinus), compound fracture, osteomyelitis of the skull, or a penetrating head wound.

Cerebral aneurysm (ruptured). Occa-

sionally, generalized seizures occur with an aneurysm rupture and reflect meningeal irritation. Associated findings commonly include nuchal rigidity, back and leg pain, fever, restlessness, irritability, and blurred vision. Confusion, lethargy, stupor, or coma occurs immediately after the abrupt onset of an excruciating headache, nausea, and vomiting. Deep coma can develop with severe bleeding. Other findings depend on the site and severity of the hemorrhage and may include hemiparesis, hemisensory deficit, dysphagia, downward deviation of the eye or conjugate deviation of the eye toward the side of the lesion, gait ataxia, miotic but reactive pupils, and visual defects. The patient may have a history of hypertension or other cardiovascular disorders. He may also have a stressful life-style, smoke, or consume an excessive amount of caffeine.

Encephalitis. In most cases, seizures are an early sign of this disorder and indicate a poor prognosis. They also may occur after recovery as a result of residual damage. Accompanying findings may include a deteriorating LOC over 48 hours, possibly leading to coma; severe headache; fever; nuchal rigidity; irritability; nausea and vomiting; photophobia; focal neurologic deficits, such as hemiparesis and hemiplegia; and cranial nerve palsies, such as ptosis. The patient may have a history of exposure to a virus that often causes encephalitis, such as an arbovirus, paramyxovirus, or herpesvirus.

Epidural hemorrhage (acute). In this disorder, seizures may follow a sudden, brief loss of consciousness, a steadily decreasing LOC, and progressively severe headache. In

When your patient has a seizure

If you witness the onset of a seizure, stay with the patient. Your main concerns should be to observe the seizure and to keep the patient from harm.

Protect the patient
Place a rolled-up towel or other soft object under the patient's head to prevent injury. Also, loosen his clothing and move any sharp or hard objects out of his way. Don't try to restrain the patient or force a hard object into his mouth; you may chip his teeth or fracture his jaw. Only at the beginning of the tonic phase can you safely insert a soft object into his mouth.

If possible during the seizure, turn the patient to one side to allow secretions to drain. Otherwise, do this at the end of the clonic phase when respirations return. If they don't return, check the airway for an obstruction. Suction as necessary.

Protect the patient after the seizure by providing a safe area where he can rest. When he awakens, reassure and reorient him. Assess his vital signs and neurologic status. Document your findings and the observations you made during the seizure.

Suspect status epilepticus
If the seizure lasts longer than 5 minutes or if a second seizure occurs before the patient fully recovers from the first, suspect status epilepticus. As or-

dered, establish an airway, start an I.V. line, administer supplemental oxygen, and begin cardiac monitoring. Also, draw blood specimens for appropriate laboratory studies.

Turn the patient on his side with his head in a semi-dependent position to drain secretions and prevent aspiration. Periodically turn him to the opposite side.

If possible, check his arterial blood gas results for hypoxemia and administer oxygen by mask, adjusting the flow rate as ordered. If necessary, assist with endotracheal intubation and mechanical ventilation. You'll most likely perform these two interventions when the seizure activity slows.

To stop the seizures, administer diazepam by slow I.V. push two or three times at 10- to 20-minute intervals, as ordered. If the patient isn't known to have a seizure disorder, the doctor may order a different drug. If the patient is hypoglycemic, a 50-ml I.V. bolus of 50% dextrose may stop the seizures. If he's alcohol-dependent, a 100-mg bolus of thiamine may stop the seizures.

If the patient has been intubated, expect to insert a nasogastric tube to prevent vomiting and aspiration. However, if the patient hasn't been intubated, the doctor may forego this procedure because the nasogastric tube itself can trigger the gag reflex and cause vomiting.

30% to 40% of patients, the brief loss of consciousness is followed by a lucid period. Associated findings in this disorder may include the following signs and symptoms: nausea and vomiting, hemiparesis, hemiplegia, high fever, ipsilateral pupil dilation, and other evidence of increasing ICP. Typically, the pa-

tient has sustained head trauma in the last 24 hours.

Hypertensive encephalopathy. A patient with this disorder may experience seizures. Other signs and symptoms may include markedly elevated blood pressure, progressively decreasing LOC (possibly leading to coma), intense headache, vomiting, visual disturbances, transient paralysis, and, eventually, Cheyne-Stokes respirations. The patient's history may reveal noncompliance with a prescribed antihypertensive regimen or a recent hypertensive crisis. Other possible causes include acute glomerulonephritis or pregnancy-induced hypertension.

Hypoglycemia. Generalized seizures commonly follow a precipitous drop in blood glucose levels. Earlier signs and symptoms include palpitations, anxiety, blurred or double vision, motor weakness, hemiplegia, trembling, excessive diaphoresis, tachycardia, myoclonic twitching, and decreasing LOC. The patient may have a history of insulin overdose, prolonged fasting, or insulin dumping syndrome following GI surgery.

Hyponatremia. Seizures may occur if serum sodium levels fall below 115 mEq/liter. Earlier signs and symptoms commonly include anxiety, irritability, headache, fatigue, postural hypotension, muscle twitching and weakness, oliguria or anuria, cold and clammy skin, poor skin turgor, weak and thready pulse, and an altered LOC ranging from lethargy to coma. Excessive thirst, tachycardia, nausea, vomiting, and abdominal cramps also may occur. The patient's history may include profuse sweating, diarrhea, or vomiting; excessive water intake; excessive infusion of dextrose in water; diuretic therapy; or overuse of tap water enemas. Other possible causes include malnutrition, extensive burns or wound drainage, adrenal insufficiency, syndrome of inappropriate antidiuretic hormone secretion, and renal disease.

Increased ICP. As ICP increases, seizures and pupillary changes may accompany gradual or sudden changes in LOC. Early signs of increased ICP include elevated blood pressure, tachycardia, altered mentation, headache, and, possibly, projectile vomiting. Later, bradycardia, widening pulse pressure, tachypnea, and apneustic and Cheyne-Stokes respirations may develop. The patient's history may reveal systemic infection, head trauma, brain tumor, or underlying metabolic or cardiac disease.

Intracerebral hemorrhage (acute). With this disorder, seizures may occur along with a severe, generalized headache and a rapid, steady drop in LOC—often progressing to coma. Hypertension and, occasionally, nuchal rigidity and vomiting also may occur. Accompanying signs and symptoms depend on the size and location of the hemorrhage and may include dizziness, nausea, decreased sensations, irregular respirations, positive Babinski's reflex, decorticate or decerebrate posturing, hemiplegia, hemiparesis, abnormal pupil size and response, aphasia, homonymous hemianopia, visual field defects, blindness, urinary incontinence, dysphagia, and dysarthria. The patient's history may include a cerebral aneurysm or congenital vascular defects, hemorrhagic disorders, hypertension, head trauma, blood dyscrasias, or anticoagulant therapy.

Lead poisoning. Seizures develop late in lead-induced encephalopathy. They follow a rapidly decreasing LOC that eventually progresses to stupor and coma. Other common early signs develop gradually and include anorexia, apathy, lethargy, malaise, anemia, behavioral disturbances, clumsiness, developmental deterioration, and persistent, forceful vomiting. An adult patient may have peripheral neuropathies and lead lines along the gums. The patient's history will include exposure to or ingestion of lead—for instance, in illegally produced alcohol or paint containing lead.

Meningitis. Severe meningitis commonly produces seizures accompanied by confusion, irritability, and possibly, stupor or coma. The disorder also causes a sudden severe, constant, generalized headache that worsens with movement; nuchal rigidity; and possibly fever. Associated findings may include chills, positive Kernig's and Brudzinski's signs, hyperreflexia, and possibly opisthotonos. As ICP increases, vomiting and occasionally papilledema develop. Other findings may include ocular palsies, facial muscle weakness, and hearing loss. The patient may have a history of systemic or sinus infection, recent dental work, or exposure to a bacterium or virus that commonly causes meningitis. These include *Haemophilus influenzae, Streptococcus pneumoniae, Neisseria meningitidis,* an enterovirus, or a paramyxovirus.

Myxedema coma. If untreated, chronic hypothyroidism can produce seizures and a decreased LOC that may lead to deep coma. Other signs and symptoms of myxedema coma include severe hypothermia, respiratory depression, hypotension, bradycardia, hypoactive reflexes, and periorbital and peripheral edema. The patient, who's typically elderly, may have a history of chronic hypothyroidism, exposure to cold, trauma, infection, or use of CNS depressants.

Pregnancy-induced hypertension. Generalized seizures are a hallmark of eclampsia—the late stage of this disorder. Early signs of preeclampsia include generalized edema and sudden weight gain of more than 3 lb a week during the second trimester or more than 1 lb a week during the third trimester. With severe preeclampsia, you'll usually note oliguria, elevated blood pressure, dizziness, diplopia, blurred vision, epigastric pain, nausea, vomiting, irritability, decreased LOC, hyperactive deep tendon reflexes, and a severe frontal headache. The patient may have a history of excessive weight gain or peripheral edema during the pregnancy or a similar episode in a previous pregnancy.

Reye's syndrome. Along with seizures, this syndrome produces hyperexcitability followed by severe, repetitive vomiting; fever; and lethargy, stupor, and coma. Signs and symptoms commonly develop over several days following a viral illness. The patient, typically a child, will have a history of recent influenza (particularly type B) or varicella, possibly with aspirin use during the infection.

Subarachnoid hemorrhage. In this disorder, seizures may be accompanied by a sudden, violent headache and an altered LOC that may progress rapidly to coma. Related findings commonly include nuchal rigidity, nausea and vomiting, dizziness, hypertension, and ipsilateral pupil dilation. The patient also may have positive Kernig's and Brudzinski's signs, photophobia, blurred vision, and possibly a fever. Focal neurologic deficits—hemiparesis, hemiplegia, sensory disturbances, and aphasia—may occur along with other signs and symptoms of increased ICP. The patient may have a history of congenital vascular defects, such as arteriovenous malformation; cardiovascular disease; smoking; excessive stress; or excessive caffeine intake.

Other causes
Generalized tonic-clonic seizures also result from certain causes that may not require immediate intervention.

Diagnostic tests. A reaction to the contrast agents used in radiologic tests may precipitate generalized seizures.

Disorders. Seizures also occur with alcohol withdrawal syndrome, arteriovenous malformation, barbiturate withdrawal, brain tumor, cerebrovascular accident, chronic renal failure, hepatic encephalopathy, hypoparathyroidism, hypoxic encephalopathy, idiopathic epilepsy, inborn errors of metabolism, intermittent acute porphyria, multiple sclerosis, neurofibromatosis, perinatal injury, sarcoidosis, and Sturge-Weber syndrome. In children, fever sometimes brings on generalized seizures.

Drugs. Toxic blood levels of aminophylline, theophylline, lidocaine, meperidine, cimetidine, and penicillins may cause generalized seizures. Use of phenothiazines, tricyclic antidepressants, amphetamines, alprostadil, isoniazid, and vincristine may cause seizures in patients with seizure disorder. Status epilepticus, marked by prolonged seizure activity or by rapidly recurring seizures with no intervening periods of recovery, most commonly is triggered by abrupt discontinuation of anticonvulsant drugs.

Skin, mottled

The term mottled skin refers to a patchy discoloration resulting from primary or secondary changes of the deep, middle, or superficial dermal blood vessels. This sign isn't always pathologic, but when it appears with other signs and symptoms, it may indicate restricted peripheral blood flow.

History questions
Explore the patient's problem by asking appropriate questions from this section.
• Did the mottling begin suddenly or gradually? What precipitated it? How long has the patient had it? Does anything make it go away?
• Does he have other symptoms, such as pain, numbness, or tingling in an arm or leg? If so, do they disappear with temperature changes? If he's experiencing pain, where is it, how long has he had it, and how severe is it? Does anything aggravate or alleviate it?
• Does the patient have cardiovascular disease? How about a condition that may predispose him to hypovolemic shock?

Physical examination
Base your assessment of the patient on the health history information you've collected.

Inspection. Observe the patient's skin color, noting the distribution of mottling as well as any pallor or diaphoresis. Evaluate his skin integrity, muscle appearance, and hair distribution, too.

Now, assess the patient's level of consciousness (LOC), noting alterations such as restlessness, confu-

Using a Doppler ultrasound probe

Palpating peripheral pulses in the legs can be difficult, especially in patients with peripheral vascular disease. To confirm whether a patient's pulse is truly absent, use a Doppler ultrasound probe — a device that intensifies the sound of blood flowing through the veins and arteries.

First, coat the pulse site with water-soluble jelly. Then turn on the machine and place the Doppler probe on the skin. Slowly move the probe around until you hear a regular swooshing sound. (Don't confuse the hum of venous flow with the swooshing of arterial flow.) Once you locate the swooshing sound, turn up the volume. Then mark the area with an X to aid subsequent assessments. If the patient has a complete arterial obstruction, you won't hear arterial sounds.

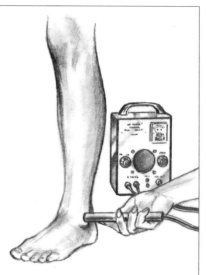

sion, or stupor. Also, observe his respiratory rate and depth. Does he have difficulty breathing? Do you note abnormal respiratory patterns?

Measure the patient's abdominal girth, then monitor for any increases. Also, monitor his urine output to detect oliguria or anuria.

Palpation. Palpate the arms and legs to assess skin texture and detect swelling and temperature differences. Check peripheral pulses, noting rate, rhythm, and intensity. If they're hard to detect, use a Doppler probe (see *Using a Doppler ultrasound probe*). Then palpate the abdomen for a pulsating epigastric mass, tenderness, or rigidity.

Percussion. Gently percuss the abdominal quadrants, noting any abnormal sounds.

Auscultation. Listen for bowel sounds, noting decreased or absent sounds. Then auscultate over the abdominal aorta to detect a systolic bruit. Be sure to monitor blood pressure and pulse pressure.

Life-threatening causes
Your assessment may lead you to suspect one or more of the following.

Abdominal aortic aneurysm (dissecting). Mottled skin below the waist accompanied by weak or absent femoral or pedal pulses characterize this acute disorder. Typically, the patient appears confused and restless, and his skin is cool and clammy. He may experience persistent abdominal and back pain, weakness, sweating, tachycardia, and dyspnea. Other common findings include increasing abdominal girth, abdominal rigidity, and a systolic bruit. On palpation, you may detect tenderness over the area of the aneurysm and an epigastric mass that pulsates before the rupture but not after it. The patient may have a history of smoking and claudication as well as other symptoms of cardiovascular disease.

Shock. Mottling that begins at the knees and elbows and progressively becomes more generalized is a late sign of shock caused by compensatory vasoconstriction. The mottling is typically preceded by restlessness, thirst, tachypnea, and slight tachycardia. Other early signs include sudden onset of pallor and cool skin in cardiogenic and hypovolemic shock or warm skin in septic shock. As shock progresses, associated findings include a rapid, thready pulse; hypotension; narrowed pulse pressure; decreased urine output; subnormal temperature; confusion; and decreased LOC. The patient's history likely will reveal a disorder that predisposes him to shock — such as massive bleeding, left ventricular failure, or septicemia.

Other causes

Mottled skin also results from conditions that may not require immediate intervention. These include acrocyanosis, arteriosclerosis obliterans, Buerger's disease, cryoglobulinemia, idiopathic or primary livedo reticularis, periarteritis nodosa, polycythemia vera, rheumatoid arthritis, and systemic lupus erythematosus. Prolonged immobility may cause bluish, asymptomatic mottling, most noticeably in dependent limbs.

Mottled skin also may be a normal reaction, such as the diffuse mottling (cutis marmorata) that occurs when exposure to cold causes venous stasis in cutaneous blood vessels. Prolonged thermal exposure — from a heating pad or hot water bottle, for example — may cause erythema ab igne, a localized, reticulated, brown-to-red mottling.

Tachycardia

Easily detected by assessing the apical, carotid, or radial pulse, tachycardia is a heart rate greater than 100 beats/minute in adults, and higher in children. Usually, the patient also complains of palpitations or of his heart "racing." A common sign, tachycardia normally results from emotional or physical stress, such as excitement, exercise, pain, and fever. Stimulants such as tobacco and caffeine can also cause this sign.

More important, however, tachycardia can be an early sign of a life-threatening disorder, such as cardiogenic or septic shock. It also may result from cardiovascular, respiratory, or metabolic disorders; electrolyte imbalances; and certain drugs, tests, and treatments. (See *What happens in tachycardia,* page 170.)

History questions

Explore the patient's problem by asking appropriate questions from this section.
• Did the patient feel palpitations when the tachycardia began? If so, has he had palpitations before? How were they treated?
• Is the patient dizzy or short of breath? Weak or fatigued? Is he experiencing chest pain? A feeling of impending doom? Severe itching

What happens in tachycardia

Tachycardia represents the heart's effort to deliver more oxygen to body tissues by increasing the rate at which blood passes through the vessels. This sign may result from overstimulation within the sinoatrial node, the atrium, the atrioventricular node, or the ventricles.

You'll recall that cardiac output is equal to heart rate (the number of contractions per minute) times stroke volume (the ventricular output for each contraction). Thus, tachycardia can lower cardiac output by reducing ventricular filling time and thus stroke volume.

As cardiac output plummets, arterial pressure and peripheral perfusion decrease. Tachycardia further aggravates myocardial ischemia by increasing the heart's demand for oxygen while reducing the duration of diastole—the period of greatest coronary artery blood flow.

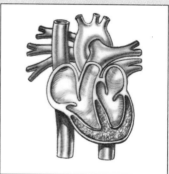

Normally, ventricular volume reaches 120 to 130 ml during diastolic filling.

In tachycardia, decreased ventricular volume leads to hypotension and decreased peripheral perfusion.

of the hands and feet? Any nausea and vomiting, diarrhea, light-headedness, cold or heat intolerance, visual disturbances, or excessive thirst, appetite, or urine output? If he has any of these signs or symptoms, ask when they began. Also, have him describe them and tell you if anything aggravates or alleviates them.

• If the patient is a woman, is she pregnant or in the postpartum period? Is she amenorrheic? If she's pregnant, has she had a sudden weight gain?

• Has the patient been exposed to allergens or organisms known to cause respiratory infections? Has he recently experienced a pulmonary or systemic injury that could predispose him to adult respiratory distress syndrome (ARDS) or shock? Also, ask about recent episodes of excessive fluid intake or loss—for instance, from wound or burn drainage or diuretic therapy.

• Does the patient have a history of trauma, diabetes, or cardiac, pulmonary, or thyroid disorders? If the patient is a child, note a history of rhinitis, fever, malaise, or anorexia. Obtain a drug history.

Physical examination

Base your assessment of the patient on the health history information you've collected.

Inspection. Observe the rate, rhythm, and quality of the patient's respirations. Keep in mind that respiratory rate and other vital signs will be different for children (see *Guide to normal pediatric vital signs,* page 172). Note whether the patient has any difficulty breathing. Check for asymmetrical chest wall movement, accessory muscle use, stridor, hoarseness, or abnormal respiratory patterns. Note whether he has a cough. If he has a productive cough, describe the sputum.

Next, inspect the patient's skin for pallor, cyanosis, poor turgor, and evidence of trauma. Assess his nail beds for decreased capillary refill time (greater than 2 seconds) and pulsations. Be sure to observe for jugular vein distention, an enlarged thyroid, tracheal deviation, and exophthalmos.

Evaluate the patient's level of consciousness (LOC), noting decreased mental acuity, restlessness, anxiety, disorientation, or confusion. Also, note any seizures.

Monitor the patient's urine output for oliguria or anuria.

Palpation. Gently palpate the eyeballs for softness and the neck for evidence of tracheal deviation or thyroid enlargement. Also, palpate over the chest and sternum for subcutaneous or bony crepitus. Check the patient's arms and legs for peripheral edema and palpate his peripheral pulses to assess rate, rhythm, and intensity.

Percussion. Next, percuss over the lungs, noting dullness, hyperresonance, or tympany. To help detect hepatomegaly, percuss the abdomen.

Auscultation. Listen over the heart for murmurs, gallops, and pericardial friction rubs. Then auscultate over the lungs, noting any abnormal sounds.

To detect orthostatic hypotension, check the patient's blood pressure with him supine and sitting. Monitor his blood pressure and pulse pressure.

Life-threatening causes

Your assessment may lead you to suspect one or more of the following.

Adult respiratory distress syndrome. In this disorder, tachycardia typically follows acute dyspnea and tachypnea. Other common findings include restlessness, grunting respirations, accessory muscle use, cyanosis, anxiety, decreased mental acuity, crackles, and rhonchi. Severe ARDS can produce signs of shock, such as hypotension and cool, clammy skin. Typically, the patient has no history of cardiac or pulmonary disease but has sustained a recent pulmonary or systemic insult.

Anaphylactic shock. Tachycardia, a dramatic drop in blood pressure, and a narrowed pulse pressure develop either within minutes or within 24 hours of exposure to an allergen, such as penicillin or an insect sting. Typically, the patient appears extremely restless and has severe pruritus, perhaps with a feeling of impending doom and a pounding headache. Later, he may develop flushing, cardiac dysrhythmias, seizures, coughing, sneezing,

Guide to normal pediatric vital signs

Use this chart when evaluating your pediatric patient's vital signs. These values are normal for a child at rest.

AGE	RESPIRATORY RATE/ MINUTE		BLOOD PRESSURE (mm Hg)		PULSE RATE/ MINUTE	
	Girls	Boys	Girls	Boys	Girls	Boys
Neonate	28	30	—	—	130	130
2 years	26	28	98/60	96/60	110	110
4 years	25	25	98/60	96/60	100	100
6 years	24	24	98/64	98/62	100	100
8 years	24	22	104/68	102/68	90	90
10 years	22	23	110/72	110/72	90	90
12 years	20	20	114/74	112/74	90	85
14 years	18	16	118/76	120/76	85	80
16 years	16	16	120/78	124/78	80	75

difficulty breathing, nasal congestion, stridor and hoarseness, nausea, abdominal cramps, and urinary and fecal incontinence. The patient may have allergies or a family history of them, and he may have been exposed to a known or common allergen.

Cardiac contusion. Resulting from blunt chest trauma, cardiac contusion can cause tachycardia accompanied by hypotension, dyspnea, and intermittent, excruciating chest pain that may radiate to the neck, the jaw, or down the arm. Inspection may reveal external bruising of the chest and abdominal area.

Cardiac dysrhythmias. In some dysrhythmias, tachycardia with a regular or irregular rhythm may be accompanied by acute or gradual dyspnea, intermittent hypotension, and palpitations. The patient also may report dizziness, light-headedness, weakness, and fatigue. He may have a history of cardiac disease or of using drugs that can cause cardiac dysrhythmias — cocaine, cardiac glycosides, or certain beta blockers, for instance.

Cardiac tamponade. In this disorder, tachycardia commonly occurs with hypotension, narrowed pulse pressure, neck vein distention, and muffled heart sounds. The patient may report fever and malaise. You also may detect pulsus paradoxus, dyspnea, Kussmaul's respirations, and cyanosis. The patient's history may include recent chest trauma, pericarditis, myocardial infarction (MI), or chronic tamponade.

Cardiogenic shock. In this form of shock, tachycardia typically is accompanied by a drop in systolic pressure to less than 80 mm Hg or 30 mm Hg less than the patient's baseline. Other common findings include narrowed pulse pressure, diminished Korotkoff's sounds, peripheral cyanosis, and pale, cool, clammy skin. The patient may be restless and anxious, and later disoriented and confused. Associated signs and symptoms may include anginal pain, dyspnea, jugular vein distention, oliguria, and a weak, rapid pulse. On auscultation, you may detect tachypnea, faint heart sounds, ventricular gallop, and, possibly, a holosystolic murmur. The patient's history may include recent or previous disorders that cause left ventricular dysfunction.

Congestive heart failure. In left ventricular failure, tachycardia occurs with dyspnea, which can develop suddenly but usually does so gradually or occurs as chronic paroxysmal nocturnal dyspnea. Other signs and symptoms include fatigue, tachypnea, low or normal blood pressure, cold intolerance, orthopnea, cough, central cyanosis, ventricular or atrial gallop, bibasilar crackles, and diffuse apical impulse. You may also note dependent edema, jugular vein distention, and prolonged capillary refill time (greater than 2 seconds).

In right ventricular failure, tachycardia is accompanied by peripheral edema, ascites, jugular vein distention, peripheral cyanosis, and hepatomegaly. The patient may have a history of cardiovascular disease or previous dyspneic episodes, fatigue, weight gain, pallor or cyanosis, diaphoresis, and anxiety. His medication history may include drugs that can cause congestive heart failure (CHF), such as angiotensin-converting enzyme inhibitors, antihypertensives, beta blockers, calcium channel blockers, corticosteroids, nonsteroidal anti-inflammatory drugs, amiodarone, carbamazepine, encainide, flecainide, recombinant interferon alfa-2a, or recombinant interleukin-2.

Diabetic ketoacidosis. Osmotic diuresis and dehydration cause tachycardia along with low blood pressure, decreased pulse pressure, and a characteristic flushed face. Accompanying signs and symptoms may include abdominal pain and distention, nausea and vomiting, Kussmaul's respirations, seizures, and stupor possibly progressing to coma. Typically, the patient reports polydipsia, polyuria, polyphagia, weight loss, fruity breath odor, and weakness persisting for several days. His history may reveal diabetes mellitus.

Epiglottitis. In this pediatric disorder, tachycardia is accompanied by dyspnea, inspiratory stridor, accessory muscle use, decreased breath sounds, high fever, drooling, and dysphagia. The child may be anxious and have a sore throat and a muffled voice. Later, he may develop cyanosis from hypoxemia that results when the swollen epiglottis obstructs the airway. His history may include exposure to *Haemophilus influenzae* type B pneumococci, or group A streptococci.

Flail chest. Multiple rib fractures produce tachycardia along with characteristic sudden dyspnea, paradoxical chest movement, severe chest pain, hypotension, tachypnea, and cyanosis. You'll note bruising and decreased or absent breath sounds over the affected side. The patient's history will include blunt chest trauma, perhaps from cardiopulmonary resuscitation.

Hyperosmolar hyperglycemic nonketotic coma. Tachycardia occurs with a drop in blood pressure, which can be dramatic if the patient loses a significant amount of fluid from osmotic diuresis. A rapidly deteriorating LOC may be accompanied by polyuria, polydipsia, weight loss, fever, shallow respirations, poor skin turgor, and, occasionally, focal or generalized tonic-clonic seizures. The patient's history may include diabetes mellitus, most commonly Type II.

Hypertensive encephalopathy. This disorder is characterized by tachycardia, tachypnea, and extremely high blood pressure (systolic pressure exceeding 200 mm Hg, diastolic pressure exceeding 120 mm Hg). Typically, the patient experiences severe headache, vomiting, seizures, visual disturbances, and transient paralysis. Eventually, he develops Cheyne-Stokes respirations and a decreased LOC that may progress to coma. The patient's history may include noncompliance with a prescribed antihypertensive regimen, a recent hypertensive crisis, acute glomerulonephritis, or pregnancy-induced hypertension.

Hyponatremia. This electrolyte imbalance produces tachycardia as well as several other signs and symptoms. You may note anxiety, orthostatic hypotension, headache, muscle twitching and weakness, fatigue, oliguria or anuria, cold and clammy skin, decreased skin turgor, irritability, lethargy, a thready pulse, and a decreased LOC possibly progressing to coma. Excessive thirst, nausea, vomiting, and abdominal cramps also may occur. Seizures commonly develop when serum sodium levels fall below 115 mEq/liter. The patient's history may include a fluid imbalance resulting from profuse sweating, diarrhea, or vomiting; excessive water intake; excessive infusion of dextrose in water; diuretic therapy; overuse of tap water enemas; malnutrition; extensive burns or wound drainage; adrenal insufficiency; syndrome of inappropriate antidiuretic hormone secretion; or renal disease.

Hypovolemic shock. Slight tachycardia that increases as blood volume decreases is an early sign of shock from blood volume loss. This sign may be accompanied by tachypnea, restlessness, thirst, and pale, cool skin. As shock progresses, systolic pressure falls to less than 80 mm Hg or to 30 mm Hg less than the patient's baseline, causing orthostatic pressure changes, diminished Korotkoff's sounds, and narrowed pulse pressure. The patient's skin becomes clammy and his pulse increasingly rapid and thready. He also may experience light-headedness, irritability, anxiety, and a decreased LOC. Other associated signs and symptoms may include anginal pain (in patients with coronary artery disease), diaphoresis, hypothermia, decreased capillary refill time (greater than 2 seconds), oliguria, and peripheral cyanosis.

Laryngotracheobronchitis. This pediatric disorder produces tachycardia with a harsh, barking cough, accessory muscle use, restlessness, anxiety, and stridor. Auscultation reveals diminished breath sounds, crackles, and rhonchi. The child may have rhinitis, fever, malaise, and anorexia for 2 to 3 days before the other symptoms appear.

Myocardial infarction. This life-threatening disorder may cause tachycardia or bradycardia. Its classic symptom, however, is crushing substernal chest pain that may radiate to the left arm, jaw, neck, abdomen, or shoulder blades. Unrelieved by rest or nitroglycerin, the chest pain may be accompanied by sudden dyspnea, pallor, clammy skin, diaphoresis, nausea, vomiting, anxiety, restlessness, weakness, dizziness, and a feeling of impending doom. The patient may develop hypotension or hypertension, an atrial gallop, murmurs, pericardial friction rub, and crackles. An MI may be the first indication of a cardiac problem, or the patient's history may reveal cardiovascular disease, hypercholesterolemia, or use of drugs that can trigger an MI — cocaine, dextrothyroxine, estramustine phosphate sodium, or recombinant interleukin-2, for example.

Pneumonia. In this disorder, tachycardia may be accompanied by sudden dyspnea, fever, shaking chills, and pleuritic chest pain that's exacerbated by deep inspiration. Depending on the stage and type of pneumonia, the patient may have a cough that produces discolored and foul-smelling sputum. Associated signs and symptoms may include decreased breath sounds, crackles, rhonchi, dull percussion sounds, whispered pectoriloquy, tachypnea, myalgias, fatigue, headache, abdominal pain, anorexia, central cyanosis, and diaphoresis. The patient's history may reveal chronic smoking, chronic obstructive pulmonary disease (COPD), or exposure to a contagious organism, hazardous fumes, or air pollution.

Pneumothorax. Life-threatening pneumothorax produces tachycardia and other signs and symptoms of distress, such as severe dyspnea, central cyanosis, and sharp chest pain that may mimic an MI. Related findings commonly include decreased or absent breath sounds with hyperresonance or tympany, subcutaneous crepitation, and decreased vocal fremitus. You also may note asymmetrical chest expansion, accessory muscle use, a nonproductive cough, tachypnea, anxiety, and restlessness. A patient with tension pneumothorax will also have tracheal deviation. His history may include recent chest trauma, subclavian vein cannulation, COPD, lung malignancy, or mechanical ventilation under pressure.

Pulmonary edema. Tachycardia and severe dyspnea commonly follow signs and symptoms of CHF, such as jugular vein distention and orthopnea. Other findings may include tachypnea, crackles in both lung fields, S_3 gallop, oliguria, a thready pulse, hypotension, diaphoresis, fatigue, recent rapid weight gain, pallor or cyanosis, and marked anxiety. The patient's cough may be dry or produce copious amounts of pink, frothy sputum. He may have a history of cardiovascular disease or previous dyspneic episodes.

Pulmonary embolism. Tachycardia typically develops after the onset of sudden dyspnea and intense anginalike or pleuritic pain that's aggravated by deep breathing and thoracic movement. You also may detect hypotension, narrowed pulse pressure, and diminished Korotkoff's sounds. Central cyanosis occurs when a large embolus obstructs pulmonary circulation. Other findings may include anxiety, tachypnea, low-grade fever, restlessness, diaphoresis, crackles, pleural friction rubs, diffuse wheezing, and dull percussion sounds. The patient's cough may be dry, or it may produce blood-tinged sputum. He also may have signs and symptoms of circulatory collapse (weak, rapid pulse and hypotension), cerebral ischemia (transient unconsciousness, coma, seizures), and hypoxia (restlessness). An elderly patient may also have hemiplegia and other focal neurologic deficits. Less common signs include massive hemoptysis (indicating pulmonary infarction), chest splinting, leg edema, and jugular vein distention. The patient's history may include varicose veins, thrombophlebitis of the deep systemic veins, hip or leg fractures, an acute MI, CHF, cardiogenic shock, congestive cardiomyopathies, recent pregnancy, or use of oral contraceptives.

Septic shock. Initially, septic shock produces tachycardia, chills, sudden fever, tachypnea, and, possibly, nausea, vomiting, and diarrhea. The patient's skin is flushed, warm, and dry; his blood pressure, normal or slightly decreased. Eventually, he may exhibit anxiety, restlessness, thirst, oliguria or anuria, and cool, clammy, cyanotic skin. As shock progresses, hypotension becomes severe (with systolic pressure dropping to less than 80 mm Hg or to 30 mm Hg less than the patient's baseline). This may be accompanied by dysrhythmias; a weak, thready pulse; decreased or absent peripheral pulses; rapid, shallow respirations; and a decreased LOC possibly progressing to coma. The patient's history may include conditions that predispose him to septic shock.

Thyrotoxicosis (thyroid storm). In this acute metabolic disturbance, tachycardia occurs with a sudden rise in systolic blood pressure,

widened pulse pressure, bounding pulse, pulsations in the capillary nail beds, and palpitations. Other common findings include exophthalmos, thyroid gland enlargement, heat intolerance, exertional dyspnea, fever excceeding 100° F (37.8° C), diarrhea, dehydration, and warm, moist skin. The patient may appear nervous and emotionally unstable and show occasional outbursts of psychotic behavior. A female patient may experience oligomenorrhea or amenorrhea. A patient with latent hyperthyroidism may have a history of excessive dietary iodine intake; symptoms may recur following stressful conditions such as surgery, infections, pregnancy, or diabetic ketoacidosis.

Other causes
Tachycardia also results from certain causes that may not require immediate intervention.

Diagnostic tests. Cardiac catheterization and electrophysiologic studies may induce transient tachycardia.

Drugs. Many drugs that affect the nervous system, circulatory system, or heart muscle can cause tachycardia. Common ones include sympathomimetics, such as epinephrine; phenothiazines, such as chlorpromazine; anticholinergics, such as atropine; thyroid drugs; vasodilators, such as hydralazine and nifedipine; nitrates, such as nitroglycerin; and alpha-adrenergic blockers, such as phentolamine. Alcohol, stimulants such as caffeine and tobacco, and illicit drugs such as marijuana can also cause tachycardia.

Surgery and pacemakers. Tachycardia also may result from cardiac surgery or pacemaker malfunction or wire irritation.

Tachypnea

A common sign of cardiopulmonary disorders, tachypnea is an abnormally fast respiratory rate — 20 or more breaths/minute. You can easily detect tachypnea by counting the patient's respirations while watching his chest rise and fall or while auscultating his lungs.

Most commonly, tachypnea indicates the need to increase minute volume — the amount of air the patient breathes each minute. This danger sign may also be accompanied by an increase in tidal volume — the volume of air the patient inhales and exhales per breath — resulting in hyperventilation. (See *Understanding tachypnea.*)

What causes tachypnea? This sign can result from any condition that produces reduced arterial oxygen tension or arterial oxygen content, decreased perfusion, increased oxygen demand, increased arterial carbon dioxide tension, or acidosis. Increased oxygen demand, for instance, may stem from exertion, anxiety, pain, or fever. Typically, respirations increase by 4 breaths/minute for every 1° F rise in body temperature. Tachypnea also may result from pulmonary irritation, stretch receptor stimulation, or neurologic disorders that disrupt midbrain and pons medullary respiratory control.

When assessing a child for tachypnea, remember that the normal respiratory rate will vary with age. (See *Guide to normal pediatric vital signs,* page 172.)

History questions

Explore the patient's problem by asking appropriate questions from

Understanding tachypnea

These illustrations show the difference between normal respirations and tachypnea.

Eupnea

With normal respirations, the rate and rhythm are regular. For an adult, the normal rate is 12 to 20 breaths/minute.

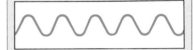

Tachypnea

An adult with tachypnea has a respiratory rate of about 20 or more breaths/minute.

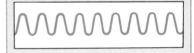

this section.

• When did the tachypnea begin? Did a specific activity or incident precede the onset? Has the patient had tachypnea before? If so, how was it treated?

• Is the patient having difficulty breathing? If so, how long has he been having difficulty? Does it get worse or better with activity? Does it get worse when he lies down?

• Is the patient experiencing associated pain? If so, how severe is it? Where is the pain and does it radiate? Find out if any activity exacerbates or alleviates the pain.

• Does the patient have other associated signs and symptoms, such as nausea, vomiting, diarrhea, diaphoresis, feelings of impending doom, fatigue, cold intolerance, anorexia, polydipsia, polyphagia, polyuria, or cough? Has he recently experi-

enced a weight loss or gain?
• Has the patient recently experienced trauma—particularly a head, abdominal, or chest injury or a leg or hip fracture? How about trauma from cardiopulmonary resuscitation? Has he had a recent systemic infection? Has he been exposed to hazardous fumes or to any organism that causes infection?
• Has the patient recently undergone any procedures that can cause pneumothorax—subclavian cannulation or mechanical ventilation under pressure, for example?
• If the patient is a woman, is she in the postpartum period?
• Does the patient's history reveal a disorder that can cause massive blood loss or one that can cause metabolic acidosis, such as diabetes mellitus or renal failure? Does the patient have a personal or family history of cardiovascular, pulmonary, or endocrine disorders?
• Does the patient have any allergies? A family history of allergies? Has he recently been exposed to a known or common allergen?
• Is the patient taking any medications that can cause congestive heart failure, such as angiotensin-converting enzyme (ACE) inhibitors or beta blockers?

Physical examination

Base your assessment of the patient on the health history information you've collected.

Inspection. Observe the patient's respirations, noting the rate and depth. Does he have difficulty breathing? Does he have abnormal respiratory patterns? Note stridor, grunting respirations, flaring nostrils, nasal congestion, use of accessory muscles, asymmetrical or paradoxical chest wall movement, and intercostal bulging or retrac-

tions. Note too whether he has a cough. If it's productive, record the color, amount, odor, and consistency of the sputum. Does the patient have an abnormal breath odor?

Assess level of consciousness (LOC), noting such alterations as restlessness, lethargy, stupor, seizures, or coma. Then check for jugular vein distention. Observe the skin for bruising or other signs of trauma, pallor or cyanosis (a late sign of hypoxemia), edema, poor skin turgor, warmth or coolness, and any rash or intense itching. Note prolonged capillary refill time (greater than 2 seconds). Monitor urine output for oliguria and anuria.

Palpation. Next, palpate the patient's peripheral pulses, noting rate, rhythm, and intensity. Gently check for a rib or sternal fracture or subcutaneous emphysema. Palpate the chest wall over the lungs for decreased tactile fremitus and decreased diaphragmatic excursion. As you palpate the abdomen, check for ascites and hepatomegaly. Assess the neck for tracheal deviation. Then gently palpate the eyeballs, noting any softness.

Percussion. Percuss over the lungs, noting hyperresonance, tympany, or dullness.

Auscultation. First, listen for abnormal breath sounds, such as crackles, rhonchi, wheezes, vocal fremitus, whispered pectoriloquy, or pleural friction rubs. Then auscultate the patient's heart sounds, noting any abnormalities—particularly murmurs or gallops.

To detect orthostatic hypotension, check the patient's blood pressure while he's supine and sitting. Then monitor his blood pressure and pulse pressure.

Life-threatening causes

Your assessment may lead you to suspect one or more of the following.

Adult respiratory distress syndrome (ARDS). Tachypnea and acute dyspnea from hypercapnia and hypoxemia are common early findings in this progressive respiratory disorder. Typical accompanying signs and symptoms include tachycardia, grunting respirations, use of accessory respiratory muscles, cyanosis, restlessness, anxiety, and decreased mental acuity. On auscultation, you'll usually detect crackles and rhonchi in both lung fields. Severe ARDS can produce signs of shock, such as hypotension and cool, clammy skin. The patient typically has no history of cardiac or pulmonary disease but has sustained recent pulmonary or systemic damage.

Airway obstruction (partial). In this obstruction, tachypnea, acute dyspnea, and inspiratory stridor occur as the patient tries to overcome the obstruction. You also may note accessory muscle use, decreased or unilaterally absent breath sounds, asymmetrical chest expansion, anxiety, cyanosis, diaphoresis, and hypotension. The patient's history may include aspiration of vomitus or a foreign body, exposure to an allergen, or a disorder causing copious respiratory secretions, such as bronchiectasis.

Anaphylactic shock. In a life-threatening allergic reaction, tachypnea from airway obstruction and hypoxemia occurs after a dramatic drop in blood pressure and narrowing of pulse pressure. Symptoms usually begin within seconds or minutes of exposure to an allergen; however, the reaction may be delayed up to 24 hours. Early symptoms include extreme restlessness, a feeling of impending doom, intense itching (especially of the hands and feet), and pounding headache. As the reaction progresses, it may produce flushing, cardiac dysrhythmias, tachycardia, seizures, coughing, sneezing, nasal congestion, stridor and hoarseness from laryngeal edema, nausea, abdominal cramps, involuntary defecation, and urinary incontinence. The patient may have allergies or a family history of allergies coupled with recent exposure to a known or suspected allergen — particularly a bee sting or a drug such as penicillin or a sulfonamide.

Asthma. During an asthma attack, tachypnea occurs as the patient struggles to inspire air through constricted airways. The patient also will have dyspnea, intercostal retraction during inspiration, intercostal bulging during expiration, accessory muscle use, and flaring nostrils. Cyanosis is a late sign of hypoxemia. On auscultation, you may note wheezing and rhonchi (or decreased breath sounds during a severe episode), tachycardia, and paradoxical pulse. When you percuss the chest, you may note hyperresonance. Palpation may reveal decreased tactile fremitus and decreased diaphragmatic excursion. The patient may have a history of asthma. Or he may have recently experienced emotional stress, been exposed to an allergen, or ingested aspirin or indomethacin.

Cardiogenic shock. In this disorder, tachypnea typically is accompanied by tachycardia, a systolic blood pressure below 80 mm Hg or 30 mm Hg lower than the patient's baseline, narrowed pulse pressure, diminished Korotkoff's sounds, peripheral cyanosis, and pale, cool, clammy skin. The patient may exhibit restlessness and anxiety, possibly progressing to disorientation and confusion. Associated signs and symptoms commonly include anginal pain, dyspnea, neck vein distention, oliguria, and a weak, rapid pulse. Auscultation may reveal faint heart sounds, a ventricular gallop, and possibly a systolic murmur. The history may include a disorder causing left ventricular dysfunction, such as myocardial infarction.

Congestive heart failure (CHF). In left ventricular failure, tachypnea results from pulmonary congestion. Dyspnea may develop suddenly but usually does so gradually or occurs as chronic paroxysmal nocturnal dyspnea. Associated signs and symptoms include fatigue, tachycardia, normal or low blood pressure, cold intolerance, orthopnea, cough, central cyanosis, weight gain, diaphoresis, and anxiety. You may detect ventricular or atrial gallop, bibasilar crackles, and a diffuse apical impulse. Dependent edema, jugular vein distention, and prolonged capillary refill time (greater than 2 seconds) also may occur.

In right ventricular failure, tachypnea typically occurs with these signs: peripheral edema, ascites, jugular vein distention, peripheral cyanosis, and hepatomegaly. The patient likely will have a history of cardiovascular disease and previous dyspneic episodes. The patient's medication history may include drugs that can precipitate CHF, such as ACE inhibitors, antihypertensives, beta blockers, calcium channel blockers, corticosteroids, nonsteroidal anti-inflammatory drugs, amiodarone, carbamazepine, doxorubicin, encainide, flecainide, recombinant interferon alfa-2a, or recombinant interleukin-2.

Diabetic ketoacidosis. When insulin isn't available to provide glucose to the body cells, metabolic acidosis produces Kussmaul's respirations (a type of tachypnea involving rapid and deep respirations). Accompanying signs and symptoms include abdominal pain and distention, nausea and vomiting, seizures, and stupor that may progress to coma. Tachycardia, hypotension, narrowed pulse pressure, and flushing result from osmotic diuresis and dehydration. Other signs and symptoms include polydipsia, polyuria, polyphagia, weight loss, fruity breath odor, and weakness persisting for several days. The patient's history may reveal Type I diabetes mellitus.

Flail chest. In this traumatic disorder, tachypnea and dyspnea result from multiple rib fractures, which may be palpable. Other findings may include paradoxical chest movement, severe chest pain, hypotension, tachycardia, and cyanosis. You may detect bruising and decreased or absent breath sounds over the affected side. The patient will have a history of blunt chest trauma or vigorous cardiopulmonary resuscitation.

Hyperosmolar hyperglycemic nonketotic coma. Tachypnea and tachycardia occur with a drop in blood pressure that may be dramatic if the patient experiences a significant fluid loss from osmotic diuresis. The patient typically experiences polyuria, polydipsia, and weight loss. You may detect fever, shallow respirations, poor skin turgor, and soft eyeballs. An altered LOC ranging from confusion to coma and, occasionally, focal or generalized tonic-clonic seizures also may occur. The patient's history may include diabetes mellitus (most commonly

Type II) and a recent stressful event, such as an infection or myocardial infarction.

Hypovolemic shock. Tachypnea and mild tachycardia that increase as blood volume decreases are early signs of hypovolemic shock. They occur when the patient becomes hypercapnic, hypoxemic, and acidotic. As shock progresses, systolic blood pressure falls below 80 mm Hg or 30 mm Hg below the patient's baseline. You may also note orthostatic blood pressure changes, diminished Korotkoff's sounds, narrowed pulse pressure, and a weak, occasionally irregular pulse. Other signs and symptoms include anginal pain (in a patient with coronary artery disease), lightheadedness, irritability, extreme thirst, diaphoresis, hypothermia, prolonged capillary refill time (greater than 2 seconds), oliguria, anxiety, restlessness, confusion, and disorientation. Peripheral vasoconstriction produces cyanosis of the limbs and pale, cool, clammy skin. The patient's history will reveal a source of blood volume loss.

Increased intracranial pressure (ICP). When ICP affects the brain stem, you may note central neurogenic hyperventilation—a form of tachypnea marked by rapid, even, deep respirations. Seizures and pupillary changes may mark a gradual or sudden change in the patient's LOC. Early signs of increased ICP include hypertension, tachycardia, altered mentation, headache, and possibly projectile vomiting. Bradycardia, widening pulse pressure, and apneustic or cluster respirations indicate deteriorating brain function. The patient's history may include any of the following: a systemic infection, head trauma,

brain tumor, or underlying metabolic or cardiac disease.

Metabolic acidosis. In this acid-base imbalance, Kussmaul's respirations (a type of tachypnea) can occur abruptly or gradually depending on the underlying disorder. Other signs and symptoms commonly include headache, fatigue, drowsiness, decreased mental acuity, altered LOC ranging from confusion to coma, seizures, hypotension, cardiac dysrhythmias, anorexia, nausea, and vomiting. You may also note signs of the underlying disorder—for example, fruity breath in diabetic ketoacidosis or alcohol breath in alcoholic ketoacidosis. The history may reveal a procedure or condition causing bicarbonate loss, such as gastric suctioning, or a disorder producing excessive acid levels, such as diabetic ketoacidosis.

Pneumonia. In this disorder, tachypnea may occur along with sudden dyspnea, fever, shaking chills, and pleuritic chest pain exacerbated by deep inspiration. Depending on the type and stage of pneumonia, the patient will have a dry cough or one that produces discolored, foulsmelling sputum. Accompanying signs and symptoms may include decreased breath sounds, crackles, rhonchi, dull percussion sounds, whispered pectoriloquy, tachycardia, myalgia, fatigue, headache, abdominal pain, anorexia, central cyanosis, and diaphoresis. The patient's history may include heavy smoking, chronic obstructive pulmonary disease (COPD), or exposure to hazardous fumes, air pollution, or an infectious organism.

Pneumothorax. A common sign of life-threatening pneumothorax, tachypnea is typically accompanied by tachycardia and dyspnea. You may also note sudden, sharp, severe chest pain, which is commonly unilateral, rarely localized, and increases with chest movement. When located centrally and radiating to the neck, the pain may mimic that of myocardial infarction.

Breath sounds may be decreased or absent on the affected side. You may detect hyperresonance or tympany, subcutaneous crepitation, and decreased vocal fremitus. Asymmetrical chest expansion, accessory muscle use, a nonproductive cough, central cyanosis, anxiety, and restlessness may occur. In tension pneumothorax, tracheal deviation commonly accompanies these findings. The patient's history may include recent subclavian vein cannulation, COPD, lung cancer, or mechanical ventilation.

Pulmonary edema. An early sign, tachypnea occurs with severe dyspnea, often preceded by signs and symptoms of congestive heart failure, such as distended neck veins and orthopnea. Other signs and symptoms include tachycardia, crackles in both lung fields, S_3 gallop, oliguria, thready pulse, hypotension, diaphoresis, pallor or cyanosis, and marked anxiety. The patient's cough may be dry or may produce copious amounts of pink, frothy sputum. The patient may report fatigue, recent weight gain, and earlier dyspneic episodes that began either abruptly or gradually. His history may reveal cardiovascular disease.

Pulmonary embolism. Tachypnea commonly occurs in life-threatening pulmonary embolism. Classic accompanying signs and symptoms include dyspnea, hypotension with narrowed pulse pressure and diminished Korotkoff's sounds, and intense angina-like or pleuritic pain that's aggravated by deep breathing and thoracic movement. Central cyanosis occurs when a large embolus significantly obstructs pulmonary circulation.

Other findings may include tachycardia, a nonproductive cough or one that produces blood-tinged sputum, low-grade fever, anxiety, restlessness, diaphoresis, crackles, pleural friction rubs, diffuse wheezing, dullness on lung percussion, signs of circulatory collapse (such as a weak, rapid pulse and hypotension), signs of cerebral ischemia (such as syncope, coma, or seizures), and — particularly in elderly patients — hemiplegia and other focal neurologic deficits. Less common signs include massive hemoptysis from a pulmonary infarction, chest splinting, leg edema, and distended neck veins. The patient's history may include varicose veins, thrombophlebitis of the deep systemic veins, hip or leg fractures, acute myocardial infarction, CHF, cardiogenic shock, congestive cardiomyopathies, recent pregnancy, or oral contraceptive use.

Septic shock. Initially, septic shock produces tachypnea along with tachycardia, fever and chills, and possibly nausea, vomiting, and diarrhea. In late stages, severe hypotension (systolic blood pressure below 80 mm Hg or 50 to 80 mm Hg less than the patient's baseline) may be accompanied by tachycardia; a weak, thready pulse; decreased or absent peripheral pulses; rapid, shallow respirations; a decreased LOC possibly progressing to coma; pale skin; cyanotic arms and legs; oliguria or anuria from decreased cardiac output; and dysrhythmias. The patient's history may include a condition predisposing him to septic shock.

Other causes
Tachypnea also results from certain disorders and drug overdoses that may not require immediate intervention.

Disorders. Tachypnea typically occurs in pulmonary disorders, such as bronchiectasis, chronic bronchitis, emphysema, interstitial fibrosis, lung abscess, malignant mesothelioma, primary pulmonary hypertension, and lung, pleural, or mediastinal tumor. It also may occur in alcohol withdrawal syndrome, anemia, and any febrile illness.

Drugs. Tachypnea may result from an overdose of salicylates or theophylline.

Vision loss

Vision loss can be sudden or gradual, temporary or permanent. In some disorders, a slight vision impairment can progress to total blindness unless the patient receives an accurate diagnosis and appropriate intervention (see *Managing sudden vision loss*).

History questions
Explore the patient's problem by asking appropriate questions from this section. If the patient needs emergency care, ask the questions as you intervene.
• Does the vision loss affect one eye or both eyes? Does it affect all or part of the visual field? Did the loss occur suddenly, or has the patient's vision been steadily worsening?
• Is the vision loss associated with any pain? If so, where is it, how

EMERGENCY INTERVENTION

Managing sudden vision loss

Sudden vision loss can signal central retinal artery occlusion or acute closed-angle glaucoma—ocular emergencies that require immediate intervention. If your patient reports a sudden vision loss, immediately notify an ophthalmologist for an emergency examination, and perform these interventions as ordered.

For a patient with suspected central retinal artery occlusion, perform light massage over his closed eyelid. Increase his carbon dioxide level, as ordered, by administering a set flow of oxygen and carbon dioxide through a Venturi mask. Or have the patient rebreathe in a paper bag to retain exhaled carbon dioxide. These steps will dilate the artery and possibly restore blood flow to the retina.

For a patient with suspected acute closed-angle glaucoma, help the doctor measure intraocular pressure with a tonometer, as ordered. (You can also estimate intraocular pressure without a tonometer by placing your fingers over the patient's closed eyelid. A rock-hard eyeball usually indicates increased intraocular pressure.) Expect to administer timolol drops and I.V. acetazolamide to help decrease intraocular pressure.

severe is it, and how long has the patient had it?
• Is the patient experiencing other associated symptoms, such as photosensitivity, halo vision, blurred vision, nausea, or vomiting?
• Has the patient experienced a recent facial or eye injury? Does he have a history of eye diseases or systemic disorders that could lead to eye problems, such as hypertension or other cardiovascular diseases or diabetes mellitus or other endocrine disorders? Does he have an

infection or allergies?
• Which medications is the patient
taking?

Physical examination
Base your assessment of the patient
on the health history information
you've collected.

Inspection. Observe both eyes,
noting edema, foreign bodies, drainage, conjunctival or scleral redness,
and any evidence of trauma. Can
the patient close his eyelids completely? Check too for ptosis.

Using a flashlight, examine the
cornea and iris for scars, cloudiness,
irregularities, and foreign bodies.
Observe pupillary size, shape, and
color. Then test the patient's direct
and consensual light reflexes and
visual accommodation. To evaluate
extraocular muscle function, test the
six cardinal fields of gaze. Finally,
test visual acuity in each eye.

Palpation. Gently palpate over each
eye, noting any hardness. Palpate
over the skull to detect any obvious
fractures or puncture wounds.

Auscultation. To check for a carotid
bruit, auscultate over the neck
and temple. Auscultate too over the
patient's closed eyes.

Vision-threatening causes
Your assessment may lead you to
suspect one or more of the following.

Glaucoma (acute closed-angle). If
left untreated, an acute episode can
lead to total blindness within 3 to
5 days. Early signs and symptoms,
which may develop quickly, include
severe eye pain, blurred vision,
halo vision, photophobia, redness of
the affected eye, a cloudy cornea,
a rock-hard eyeball, a swollen upper
eyelid, and a moderately dilated,

fixed pupil. Increased intraocular
pressure may cause headache, nausea, and vomiting. The patient
may have a history of chronic glaucoma, elevated intraocular pressure,
or progressively blurred vision.
(For more information, see *What
causes sudden vision loss.*)

Ocular trauma. Sudden unilateral or
bilateral vision loss may occur after
an eye injury. The vision loss may
be total or partial, permanent or
temporary. The eyelids may be
reddened, edematous, and lacerated.
Intraocular contents may be ex-
truded.

Retinal artery occlusion (central). In
this painless ocular emergency,
sudden unilateral vision loss may be
partial or complete. If untreated,
this disorder may progress to permanent blindness within hours. The
patient will have a sluggish direct
pupillary response and a normal
consensual response. His history
may include atherosclerosis, infection, embolic disease, or a condition
causing reduced ocular blood flow—
temporal arteritis, carotid occlusion,
or low output cardiac failure, for
example.

Other causes
Vision loss also results from certain
causes that may not require immediate intervention.

Disorders. Vision loss can result
from numerous ocular disorders, including amblyopia, amaurosis fugax
(transient monocular blindness),
cataract formation, diabetic retinopathy, endophthalmitis, hereditary
corneal dystrophies, keratitis, optic
nerve glioma, optic neuritis, retinal
detachment, retinal vein occlusion,
retinitis pigmentosa, retinoblastoma,
retrolental fibroplasia, senile macu-

PATHOPHYSIOLOGY

What causes sudden vision loss

Sudden vision loss may result from acute closed-angle glaucoma or central retinal artery occlusion. Here's how these two disorders cause blindness.

Acute closed-angle glaucoma

In a normally functioning eye, the ciliary body produces aqueous humor, which flows from the posterior to the anterior chamber, then through the trabecular meshwork to the canal of Schlemm (outflow channel). From there it travels into the venous circulation.

When the iris comes in contact with the trabecular meshwork, this flow is blocked, causing a sudden increase in intraocular pressure—acute closed-angle glaucoma. The resulting compromise in the optic nerve's blood supply can lead to blindness.

Central retinal artery occlusion

In a patient who has this disorder secondary to atherosclerosis or heart disease, emboli dislodge from the carotid artery or heart valves and travel into the retinal artery, occluding it. For a short time, the retina still receives blood from the choriocapillaries, which are attached to Bruch's membrane. So the retina survives for a while.

But it needs the full flow of the central retinal artery—its major blood supply. If this flow isn't restored in 2 hours, the retina becomes edematous and necrotic.

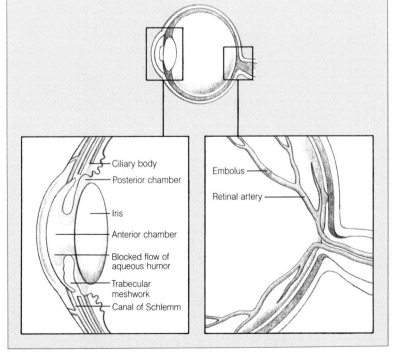

Ciliary body
Posterior chamber
Iris
Anterior chamber
Blocked flow of aqueous humor
Trabecular meshwork
Canal of Schlemm

Embolus
Retinal artery

lar degeneration, trachoma, uveitis, and vitreous hemorrhage. Other possible causes include cerebrovascular accident, concussion, congenital rubella, congenital syphilis, herpes zoster, Marfan's syndrome, pituitary tumor, Stevens-Johnson syndrome, and temporal arteritis.

Drugs. Chloroquine therapy may cause gradual vision loss, which may continue even after therapy stops. Prolonged use causes irreversible vision loss. Phenylbutazone may cause vision loss and increased susceptibility to retinal detachment. Corticosteroids, digitalis derivatives, indomethacin, ethambutol, lithium, quinine sulfate, and methanol toxicity also may cause vision loss.

Wheezing

Adventitious breath sounds, wheezes may be described as having a high-pitched, musical, squealing, creaking, or groaning quality. When originating in the large airways, they can be heard by placing your ear over the patient's chest wall or mouth. When originating in the smaller airways, wheezes can be heard by auscultating the anterior or posterior chest wall. Unlike crackles and rhonchi, wheezes can't be cleared by coughing.

Usually, prolonged wheezing occurs during expiration when the bronchi are narrowed. Causes of airway narrowing include bronchospasm; mucosal thickening or edema; partial obstruction from a tumor, a foreign body, or secretions; and extrinsic pressure, as from a tumor or goiter. With an airway obstruction, wheezing occurs during inspiration and is known as *stridor*.

History questions
Explore the patient's problem by asking appropriate questions from this section.
• When did the wheezing begin? Was the onset associated with a specific incident? Has the patient experienced a similar episode before? If so, was the precipitating incident the same? What alleviated the symptoms?
• Is he dyspneic? If so, when did the dyspnea begin? Does it worsen at night or when he lies down?
• Does the patient have associated pain? If so, when did it start, where is it, how severe is it, and how long has he had it? Does the pain radiate or increase with breathing, coughing, or position changes?
• If he has a cough, when did it start? Is it paroxysmal? Productive? If so, have him describe the sputum color and consistency.
• What about other accompanying symptoms, such as intense itching, nausea, abdominal cramps, nasal congestion, or sneezing?
• Has the patient recently experienced trauma, particularly a hip or leg fracture? Does he have cancer — especially of the lungs or thoracic cage? If the patient is a woman, is she pregnant or in the postpartum period?
• Does the patient or family member have asthma or allergies? Has the patient recently been exposed to a known or common allergen? Does he smoke? Has the patient been exposed to substances that would predispose him to pulmonary disease or lung cancer? Ask too about activities that would predispose him to thrombophlebitis.
• Does the patient have a history of pulmonary, cardiovascular, endocrine, or autoimmune disorders?
• Which medications is the patient taking?

Physical examination

Base your assessment of the patient on the health history information you've collected.

Inspection. Observe the patient's respirations, noting rate and depth. Does he have difficulty breathing or abnormal respiratory patterns? Note any wheezing or stridor.

As the patient breathes, inspect his chest for accessory muscle use, increased or paroxysmal chest wall motion, and intercostal, suprasternal, or supraclavicular retractions or bulging. Also look for nasal flaring. Observe his chest for an abnormality that could indicate chronic lung disease, such as barrel chest.

Next, assess the patient's level of consciousness (LOC), noting such alterations as restlessness, anxiety, seizures, stupor, or coma. Also look for neurologic deficits, such as hemiplegia or focal deficits.

If the patient has a cough, note the characteristics of any produced sputum. Finally, inspect the skin for diaphoresis or cyanosis and the neck for jugular vein distention.

Palpation. Check the patient's peripheral pulses for rate, rhythm, and intensity. Also, palpate over the lungs, noting decreased tactile and vocal fremitus or decreased diaphragmatic excursion.

Percussion. Next, percuss over the lungs, noting any areas of dullness or hyperresonance.

Auscultation. Listen to determine when in the respiratory cycle wheezing occurs. Note any adventitious breath sounds, such as decreased or absent sounds, crackles, rhonchi, or pleural friction rubs. Auscultate the heart for abnormal heart sounds, gallops, or murmurs.

Monitor the patient's blood pressure and pulse pressure. Note the intensity of Korotkoff's sounds and check for a paradoxical pulse.

Life-threatening causes

Your assessment may lead you to suspect one or more of the following.

Airway obstruction (partial). Sudden stridor, tachypnea, and acute dyspnea occur as the patient tries to overcome a severe obstruction (defined as at least a 75% decrease in the upper airway's cross-sectional diameter). The patient also may have such signs and symptoms as expiratory wheezing, accessory muscle use, decreased or unilaterally absent breath sounds, asymmetrical chest expansion, anxiety, cyanosis, diaphoresis, and hypotension. His history may include aspiration of vomitus or a foreign body (such as bone, teeth, or blood in a trauma victim), exposure to an allergen, or a disorder producing copious secretions.

Anaphylactic shock. Stridor and possibly expiratory wheezing resulting from laryngeal edema occur late in this disorder. Early findings include tachypnea, extreme restlessness, a feeling of impending doom, intense itching (especially of the hands and feet), pounding headache, a dramatic drop in blood pressure, and narrowed pulse pressure. In most cases, signs and symptoms occur seconds to minutes after exposure to an allergen; however, delayed reactions of up to 24 hours may occur. As the reaction progresses, you may note flushing, cardiac dysrhythmias, tachycardia, seizures, coughing, sneezing, nasal congestion, nausea, abdominal cramps, and fecal and urinary incontinence. The patient may have

EMERGENCY INTERVENTION

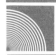

Managing acute asthma

If your assessment findings indicate that your patient is having an acute asthma attack, take these steps.

Initial interventions

Help the patient into a comfortable position that enhances gas exchange—high Fowler's position, for example. Then administer humidified oxygen via a nasal cannula at a rate of 2 to 4 liters/minute. Monitor the patient's arterial blood gas and oxygen saturation levels, adjusting the flow rate accordingly. If possible, use pulse oximetry to monitor his oxygen saturation. If the doctor doesn't order specific settings and the patient doesn't have underlying pulmonary disease, you should set the oximeter's default alarms as follows:

• high saturation, 100%
• low saturation, 85%
• high pulse rate, 140
• low pulse rate, 55.

Next, begin an I.V. infusion of dextrose 5% in water to ensure adequate hydration, liquefy secretions, and aid expectoration. Once you have this infusion going, you'll also be able to administer emergency I.V. drugs, as ordered.

Monitor the patient

Now, turn your attention back to assessment. Monitor the patient for altered level of consciousness—a reliable indicator of poor tissue oxygenation. Assess his respirations and breath sounds every 15 minutes until his condition is stable. Note ineffective breathing and impaired gas exchange. Note too whether he's becoming fatigued from the work of breathing.

Administer drugs

As ordered, administer drugs to treat bronchospasm. In a young, otherwise healthy patient, subcutaneous epinephrine or theophylline may be given instead of a beta-adrenergic. In an older patient or one with cardiovascular problems, a beta$_2$-specific drug will usually be given by a metered dose inhaler or nebulizer. The reason: This drug will cause milder adverse cardiovascular effects.

You may administer a corticosteroid if that's what has helped the patient before or if the attack is severe and he doesn't respond to epinephrine or theophylline within 30 to 60 minutes. If the patient doesn't respond to any of these drugs, you may administer ipratropium by metered dose inhaler every 4 to 6 hours.

After starting drug therapy, monitor the patient for therapeutic and adverse reactions. If the doctor prescribed theophylline, obtain venous blood samples for theophylline analysis. The usual therapeutic range is 10 to 20 mcg/ml. Be sure to monitor for signs and symptoms of toxicity, such as nausea, vomiting, diarrhea, tachycardia, confusion, and headaches, and for signs of a subtherapeutic dosage, such as increased wheezing and respiratory distress.

---

allergies or a family history of them along with recent exposure to a known or a common allergen—especially a bee sting or a drug such as a penicillin or sulfonamide.

Asthma. An early, cardinal sign of an acute asthma attack, wheezing can be heard at the patient's mouth during expiration. Other findings include tachypnea, dyspnea, intercostal retraction on inspiration and intercostal bulging on expiration, accessory muscle use, and flaring nostrils. Cyanosis is a late sign of hypoxemia. On auscultation, you'll hear wheezing and rhonchi or decreased breath sounds during a severe episode. You'll also note tachycardia and a paradoxical pulse. You may detect hyperresonance on chest percussion as well as decreased vocal and tactile fremitus and decreased diaphragmatic excursion on palpation. The patient may have a history of asthma, recent exposure to a known or suspected allergen, excessive emotional stress, or ingestion of aspirin or indomethacin. (For more information, see *Managing acute asthma.*)

Pulmonary edema. Mild to severe wheezing may occur during an episode of pulmonary edema. The cardinal signs — tachypnea and severe dyspnea — typically follow signs and symptoms of congestive heart failure, such as orthopnea and distended neck veins.

Other findings commonly include tachycardia, crackles in both lung fields, S_3 gallop, oliguria, a thready pulse, hypotension, diaphoresis, pallor or cyanosis, fatigue, weight gain, and marked anxiety. The patient may have a dry cough or one that produces copious pink, frothy sputum. The patient's history may include cardiovascular disease or dyspneic episodes with an abrupt or gradual onset.

Pulmonary embolism. Mild to moderate diffuse wheezing occasionally occurs in pulmonary embolism. Usually, such wheezing is more common when subsequent episodes of pulmonary embolism occur. The classic signs and symptoms include acute dyspnea, hypotension with narrowed pulse pressure and diminished Korotkoff's sounds, and intense angina-like or pleuritic pain that's aggravated by deep breathing and thoracic movement. Central cyanosis occurs when a large embolus causes a significant obstruction of the pulmonary circulation.

On auscultation, you may detect crackles and pleural friction rubs. You also may note dullness when percussing over the lungs. Other common findings include tachycardia, tachypnea, a dry cough or one that produces blood-tinged sputum, a low-grade fever, anxiety, restlessness, diaphoresis, altered LOC (ranging from syncope to coma), seizure activity, and — particularly in an elderly patient — hemiplegia and other focal neurologic deficits. Less common signs include massive hemoptysis from pulmonary infarction, chest splinting, leg edema, and distended neck veins. The patient's history may reveal a cardiovascular disorder, such as varicose veins, thrombophlebitis of the deep systemic veins, acute myocardial infarction, congestive heart failure, cardiogenic shock, or congestive cardiomyopathy; hip or leg fracture; a recent pregnancy; or use of oral contraceptives.

Other causes

Wheezing also results from conditions that may not require immediate intervention. For instance, mild to severe wheezing can occur in chronic obstructive pulmonary disorders, such as bronchiectasis, byssinosis, chronic bronchitis, emphysema, interstitial fibrosis, lung tumor, and pneumonia. Other possible causes include cystic fibrosis, inhalation injury, pulmonary tuberculosis, sarcoidosis, thoracic cage deformities, thyroid goiter, and Wegener's granulomatosis.

SUGGESTED READINGS

AHFS Drug Information 90. Bethesda, Md.: American Society of Hospital Pharmacists, 1990.

Bates, B., and Hoeckelman, R.A. *A Guide to Physical Examination and History Taking,* 4th ed. Philadelphia: J.B. Lippincott Co., 1987.

Behrman, R.E., and Vaughan, V.C., III. *Nelson Textbook of Pediatrics,* 13th ed. Philadelphia: W.B. Saunders Co., 1987.

Braunwald, E., ed. *Heart Disease: A Textbook of Cardiovascular Medicine,* 3rd ed. Philadelphia: W.B. Saunders Co., 1988.

Braunwald, E., et al., eds. *Harrison's Principles of Internal Medicine,* 11th ed. New York: McGraw-Hill Book Co., 1988.

Drug Information for the Health Care Professional, 10th ed. Rockville, Md.: United States Pharmacopeial Convention, 1990.

Kempe, C.H., et al., eds. *Current Pediatric Diagnosis and Treatment,* 9th ed. Los Altos, Calif.: Appleton & Lange, 1987.

Kinney, M.R., et al. *AACN'S Clinical Reference for Critical-Care Nursing,* 2nd ed. New York: McGraw-Hill Book Co., 1987.

Krupp, M.A., et al., eds. *Current Medical Diagnosis and Treatment,* 25th ed. Los Altos, Calif.: Appleton & Lange, 1986.

Malasanos, L., et al. *Health Assessment,* 4th ed. St. Louis: C.V. Mosby Co., 1989.

Morton, P.G. *Health Assessment in Nursing.* Springhouse, Pa.: Springhouse Corp., 1989.

Nursing91 Drug Handbook. Springhouse, Pa.: Springhouse Corp., 1991.

Signs & Symptoms Handbook. Springhouse, Pa.: Springhouse Corp., 1988.

Vaughan, D., and Asbury, T. *General Ophthalmology,* 12th ed. Los Altos, Calif.: Appleton & Lange, 1989.

SELF-TEST

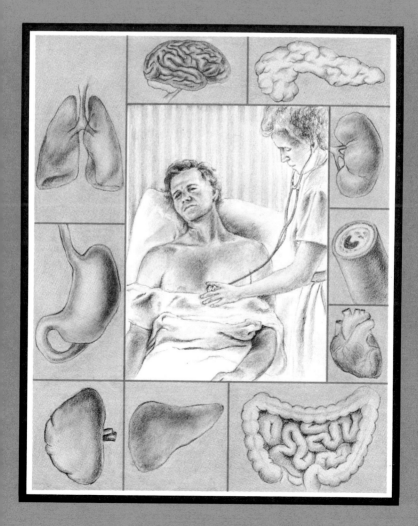

1. *Unlike somatic abdominal pain, visceral abdominal pain is:*
a. bright, sharp, and intense.
b. well localized.
c. referred from another site that has the same nerve supply.
d. a slowly developing, dull ache.

2. *You'd consider your patient to be anuric if he had:*
a. no urine output for 6 hours.
b. a urine output of less than 75 ml/24 hours.
c. a urine output of at least 200 ml/day.
d. pain and burning on urination.

3. *After discovering that your patient is apneic, you'd first:*
a. raise the head of the bed.
b. check his airway for signs of obstruction.
c. palpate his pulse.
d. auscultate his chest for breath sounds.

4. *You'd consider your patient to have absent bowel sounds if:*
a. you heard no bowel sounds after auscultating for at least 5 minutes in each abdominal quadrant.
b. you couldn't see peristaltic waves.
c. you heard no bowel sounds after auscultating for at least 1 minute in each abdominal quadrant.
d. he had nausea, vomiting, and constipation persisting for 2 days.

5. *High-pitched, tinkling, hyperactive bowel sounds accompanied by tympany and abdominal distention may indicate:*
a. hunger.
b. mechanical intestinal obstruction.
c. appendicitis.
d. a drug allergy.

6. *You'd become concerned if a patient who'd suffered a serious head injury developed bradycardia and:*
a. decreased urine output.
b. headache.
c. widening pulse pressure and tachypnea.
d. diaphoresis.

7. *Which of the following respiratory rates would indicate bradypnea in a 2-year-old child?*
a. 35 breaths/minute
b. 30 breaths/minute
c. 25 breaths/minute
d. 20 breaths/minute

8. *Excruciating, tearing, stabbing chest pain that begins suddenly would typically be associated with:*
a. myocardial infarction.
b. dissecting aortic aneurysm.
c. pulmonary embolism.
d. pulmonary edema.

9. *Which of following is true of Cheyne-Stokes respirations? They:*
a. are rapid, shallow respirations resulting from hypoxemia.
b. occur only during sleep.
c. most commonly occur in children.
d. typically indicate disrupted respiratory regulation in the brain stem.

10. *The term* Turner's sign *refers to:*
a. bruising over the flank.
b. bruising over the abdomen.
c. a macular rash across the scapula.
d. perineal hyperemia.

11. *Central cyanosis reflects:*
a. inadequate oxygenation of the systemic arterial blood.
b. sluggish peripheral circulation.
c. reduced oxygen saturation in the venous blood.
d. increased oxygen saturation in the arterial blood.

12. *A health history for a patient with diarrhea should include which of the following questions?*
a. Do you experience burning on urination?
b. Do you have a history of atrial fibrillation?
c. Are you taking an antibiotic drug?
d. Are you taking a diuretic drug?

13. *Dyspnea accompanied by tachycardia, fatigue, central cyanosis, distended*

neck veins, prolonged capillary refill time, and pulmonary congestion may point to:
a. acute renal failure.
b. congestive heart failure.
c. bronchitis.
d. partial airway obstruction.

14. *What's the most commonly reported neurologic symptom?*
a. headache
b. confusion
c. paresthesia
d. weakness

15. *The term* massive hematemesis *refers to:*
a. more than 1,500 ml of bloody urine output in 24 hours.
b. vomiting of bright red blood.
c. vomiting at least 500 ml of blood.
d. passing 500 ml of bright red blood rectally.

16. *To be meaningful, blood pressure readings must be:*
a. taken with the patient supine.
b. repeated within 5 minutes.
c. taken with the patient standing.
d. compared to the patient's baseline blood pressure.

17. *The term* critical hyperthermia *refers to body temperature above:*
a. 106° F
b. 105° F
c. 104° F
d. 102° F

18. *Which of the following is not associated with hypotension?*
a. expanded intravascular space with normal intravascular volume
b. reduced intravascular volume
c. decreased cardiac output
d. increased intravascular volume

19. *Hypothermia can be life-threatening because:*
a. the body loses the ability to regulate temperature.
b. shivering increases the body's metabolic demands.
c. cerebral anoxia occurs.
d. myocardial ischemia occurs.

20. *Which of the following may indicate that your patient has an altered level of consciousness?*
a. an impaired ability to answer health history questions
b. a headache
c. slurred speech, ptosis, and facial droop
d. a history of alcohol abuse

21. *Oliguria is defined as:*
a. urine output greater than 1,500 ml/24 hours.
b. no urine output in 24 hours.
c. urine output less than 75 ml/24 hours.
d. urine output less than 400 ml/24 hours.

22. *Which of the following describes decorticate posturing?*
a. an abnormal flexor response that has a more favorable prognosis than decerebrate posturing
b. an abnormal extensor response that has a more favorable prognosis than decerebrate posturing
c. an abnormal flexor response that has a less favorable prognosis than decerebrate posturing
d. an abnormal extensor response that has a less favorable prognosis than decerebrate posturing

23. *Which of the following describes a correct cardiovascular assessment method for an infant or a young child?*
a. Palpate the radial pulse to determine if peripheral pulses are present.
b. Palpate the dorsal pedal or posterior tibial pulse to determine if peripheral pulses are present.
c. Palpate the brachial, popliteal, or femoral pulses to evaluate arterial circulation.
d. Perform only the capillary blanch test to evaluate arterial circulation.

24. *Pulse pressure is defined as the difference between the:*
a. apical pulse rate and systolic blood pressure.
b. apical pulse rate and diastolic blood pressure.
c. systolic blood pressure on inspiration and systolic blood pressure on expiration.
d. systolic and diastolic blood pressures.

25. When monitoring pupillary changes, you'd assess all of the following except:
a. pupil and iris color.
b. pupil size.
c. pupil reactivity to light.
d. bilateral pupil equality.

26. When a patient is having a generalized seizure, your first priority is to:
a. note when the seizure starts, how long it lasts, where in the body it starts, and where it spreads.
b. auscultate his lungs.
c. telephone his family to obtain a complete health history.
d. assess his level of consciousness.

27. If your patient develops tachycardia, you should auscultate his heart for abnormal heart sounds and:
a. his abdomen for hyperactive bowel sounds.
b. his carotid arteries for bruits.
c. his lungs for adventitious breath sounds.
d. his eyeballs for bruits.

28. Tachypnea usually indicates:
a. fever.
b. the need to increase the patient's minute volume.
c. the need to sedate the patient.
d. pulmonary disease.

29. When assessing a patient who's experienced sudden vision loss, you should ask whether he has a history or family history of:
a. bradycardia.
b. tachycardia.
c. hypertension.
d. hypotension.

30. Which of the following statements is correct? Wheezing:
a. can be cleared with coughing.
b. can't be cleared with coughing.
c. can be heard only with a stethoscope.
d. produces a sound identical to that of crackles.

ANSWERS				
1. d	**7.** d	**13.** b	**19.** a	**25.** a
2. b	**8.** b	**14.** a	**20.** a	**26.** a
3. b	**9.** d	**15.** c	**21.** d	**27.** c
4. a	**10.** a	**16.** d	**22.** a	**28.** b
5. b	**11.** a	**17.** b	**23.** c	**29.** c
6. c	**12.** c	**18.** d	**24.** d	**30.** b

INDEX

i refers to an illustration; t refers to a table

i refers to an illustration; t refers to a table

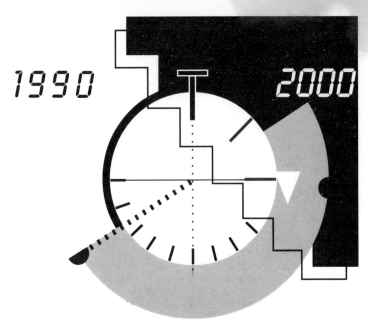

1990   2000

Nursing Magazine
In the future as in the past...

You can rely on *Nursing* magazine to keep your skills sharp and your practice current—with award—winning nursing journalism.

Each monthly issue is packed with expert advice on the legal, ethical, and personal issues in nursing, plus up-to-the-minute...

- Drug information—warnings, new uses, and approvals

- Assessment tips

- Emergency and acute care advice

- New treatments, equipment, and disease findings

- Photostories and skill sharpeners

- AIDS updates

- Career tracks and trends

SAVE 38%
Enter your subscription today.
